AGING STRONG: STRENGTH TRAINING FOR WOMEN OVER 60

EMPOWERING YOUR BODY AND MIND FOR A VIBRANT LIFE

WILLOW HALL

D1521151

TABLE OF CONTENTS

Introduction   7

1. HOW AGING AFFECTS MUSCLE MASS, BONE
DENSITY, AND OVERALL STRENGTH   11
Muscle Mass and Muscle Strength   11
Hormonal Changes   12
Bone Health   14

2. ADDRESSING COMMON MISCONCEPTIONS
ABOUT STRENGTH TRAINING IN OLDER
ADULTS   17
Strength Training Is Only for Younger People   17
Older People Are Prone to Injury From Strength
Training   18
Lifting Weights Makes Women Bulky   18
Cardiovascular Exercises Are Sufficient   19
It Is Too Late to Start Strength Training   19
Strength Training Requires a Gym Membership or
Expensive Equipment   20
Experiencing Pain and Discomfort During and After
Strength Training Is Normal   20
Only Heavy Weights Are Effective   20
Summary   21

3. OVERCOMING BARRIERS AND FEARS
ASSOCIATED WITH STRENGTH TRAINING   23
Psychological Barriers   23
Physical Barriers   25
Logistical Barriers   26
Social and Cultural Barriers   27
Educational Barriers   27
Summary   28

4. BENEFITS OF STRENGTH TRAINING FOR OLDER
WOMEN   29

5. ASSESSING CURRENT FITNESS LEVEL   33
    Tip   34
    Consulting With Your Health Care Provider   34
    Completing Self-Assessments of Your Physical
    Condition   35
    Body Composition Analysis   42

6. SETTING REALISTIC GOALS AND DESIGNING
    AN EFFECTIVE WORKOUT PROGRAM   47
    Setting Realistic Goals   48
    Designing an Effective Workout Program   50
    Seeking Professional Guidance   52
    Summary   55

7. WARM-UP MOVEMENTS   57

8. ESSENTIAL STRENGTH TRAINING EXERCISES   61
    Upper-Body exercises   62
    Lower-Body Exercises   69
    Core Exercises   75
    Modifications and Variations for Different Fitness
    Levels and Abilities   79

9. ADVANCED TRAINING TECHNIQUES   83
    Incorporating Resistance Bands, Stability Balls, and
    Other Equipment   83
    Exploring Different Training Modalities   86
    Cross-Training and Its Benefits for Overall Fitness
    and Injury Prevention   89

10. COOLDOWN MOVEMENTS   93
11. CREATING A SAFE AND SUPPORTIVE WORKOUT
    ENVIRONMENT   97

12. NUTRITION AND RECOVERY   101
    Importance of Proper Nutrition for Muscle Repair
    and Recovery   101
    Understanding Muscle Repair and Recovery   101
    Summary   108

13. HYDRATION'S ROLE IN STRENGTH TRAINING   111
    Physiological Role of Hydration   111
    Effects of Dehydration on Strength Training   112
    Optimal Hydration Strategies for Strength Training   113

14. OVERCOMING CHALLENGES AND STAYING
MOTIVATED   119
    Dealing With Age-Related Health Issues and
    Chronic Conditions   119
    Finding Support From Peers, Trainers, and Online
    Communities   122
    Setting Realistic Expectations and Celebrating
    Progress   125

15. LONG-TERM MAINTENANCE AND
SUSTAINABILITY   129
    Strategies for Maintaining Strength and Function as
    You Age   129
    Adapting Workouts to Changing Needs and Abilities 134
    Cultivating a Lifelong Commitment to Health and
    Fitness   136

16. INCORPORATING CARDIOVASCULAR AND
FLEXIBILITY EXERCISES FOR OVERALL FITNESS   139
    Creating a Balanced Routine   142
    Summary   143

    Conclusion   145
    Glossary   155
    References   159

Introduction

The Importance of Strength Training for Women Over 60

There is a negative connotation with aging, especially once you surpass a certain age, but there are also many misconceptions! Reaching a mature age, like 60, is not a death sentence; it merely means that a different approach must be taken for certain activities. It requires you to listen to your body and adjust the way you do certain things.

Aging is an unavoidable part of life; why not make the best of it?

We have long heard of many studies proving the benefits of exercise. How exercising enriches your life, lengthens life expectancy, and generally leaves you healthier, happier, and more energized (*7 Great Reasons*, 2021). While this is a truth, many believe that once you reach a certain age, you cannot exercise anymore as you become more fragile and prone to injuries due to your body slowing down, muscles deteriorating, health issues cropping up, and limited mobility.

This is untrue! Yes, adjustments will probably have to be made, but regardless of your age, you can look and feel strong by incorporating an unpopular form of exercise among the more mature population: strength training!

As bizarre as it may sound, strength training, also known as weightlifting or resistance training, is beneficial for all age groups. It also becomes increasingly important for one to implement it in their exercise routine as they grow older as it assists in the following:

- **Loss of muscle mass:** The older we get, the less muscle mass our body is able to preserve. Strength training counters this issue as it helps with muscle growth. This is important for maintaining our ability to move and function without assistance. This also reduces the risk of developing certain health problems like dementia (Volpi et al., 2004).
- **Reduced bone density:** Fragile and brittle bones are common among the elderly; thus, we regularly hear of someone falling down and then needing knee or hip surgery. Strength training stimulates bone growth, which in turn reduces the risk of bone fractures or breaks (Volpi et al., 2004).
- **Joint pain–injury:** The probability of experiencing issues related to joints, such as osteoarthritis, becomes higher with age. Hence, building up muscles that can help maintain one's mobility and day-to-day functioning is crucial to avoid joint-related injuries (Volpi et al., 2004).
- **Weight gain:** As we age, our metabolism tends to slow down. However, with strength training, the muscle mass built can help increase the metabolism, enabling the body

to burn off more calories and prevent unwanted weight gain (*What Women Need to Know*, n.d.).

- **Decline in mental health**: Mental health struggles can be faced by anyone. We all experience different situations in our lives that, if not managed, can endanger our well-being. Regular exercise, including strength training, has proven to boost one's mood and enhance mental health and overall well-being. Having a consistent routine and an outlet for your energy is also a technique to help manage some mental health problems (Barahona-Fuentes et al., 2021).

The importance of strength training cannot be emphasized enough; it is something that must be an integral part of everyone's life. The type of exercises, modifications, and repetitions will differ for each person, but it is important to integrate them into your daily life.

1. How Aging Affects Muscle Mass, Bone Density, and Overall Strength

Before we can advocate for strength training for older adults, it is necessary to address actual fears around age-related health conditions that can cause older adults to shy away.

MUSCLE MASS AND MUSCLE STRENGTH

Research has shown that some start to experience muscle mass loss from the age of 30! This decline rate worsens as the decades pass, so the muscle mass loss percentage becomes approximately 4–5% for people in their '60s. More worrying than that, muscle strength loss is 2–5 times faster than muscle mass loss, averaging about 9–10% for people in their '60s. This does not even take into consideration the impact that a sudden illness can have, further weakening muscle health. For older adults, a severe loss in muscle mass and, thus, in function can cause disability or even death.

The decline in muscle and strength mass can be due to a variety of factors, such as lowered protein intake, decreased physical activity, lowered hormone levels, chronic illnesses, insulin resistance, etc.

The rate of muscle strength loss is larger than the muscle mass loss, which is a normal part of healthy aging. The problem comes in when muscle mass and function, alongside physical ability and strength, deteriorate faster than normally expected from aging. This is called sarcopenia, it has a large impact on your quality of life, as it reduces your mobility and ability to complete normal daily tasks (Volpi et al., 2004).

HORMONAL CHANGES

At different periods of life, whether male or female, we can expect to experience age-related hormonal changes. In men, this comes in the form of decreased levels of testosterone, while in women, in the form of decreased levels of estrogen and progesterone, which is known as menopause, a period in which their menstrual cycle comes to an end, causing an end to the ovulation process and, therefore, an end to the production of eggs. This can occur between the ages of 45 and 55 and may affect each individual in different ways.

Many symptoms are associated with menopause, but we will mainly look at its impact on muscle mass. Hormonal changes due to menopause in women tend to affect their metabolism, which serves the purpose of supplying cells in the body with enough energy to fulfill their function. The main cells impacted are the connective tissues responsible for moving nutrients and other substances from one tissue to another and storing fat. Hence, the process of supplying the body with nutrients and converting fat into energy may be disturbed, leading to an excess of fat storage in the body. The blockage of nutrients moving from one cell to another, as well as the excessive storing of fat, then results in the wearing down of muscles, putting one at risk of obesity and other related chronic illnesses. When this happens, there can be a significant decline in one's ability to do everyday activities, causing them to rely on external help for support.

Aging can create a vicious cycle whereby the harm caused by hormonal changes that occur naturally with age leads to the development of chronic illnesses. As observed previously, hormonal changes can put one at risk of obesity, which, in turn, is related to chronic illnesses such as diabetes and cardiovascular diseases. If the cells in the body fail to convert food into energy, there is a high chance that one can become insulin resistant; the pancreas may produce little to no amount of a hormone called insulin, which is responsible for the regulation of blood sugar levels. This results in the infiltration of high amounts of sugar—glucose—into the bloodstream, known as diabetes. Cardiovascular diseases are also exacerbated by any damage in the blood vessels that pump blood into the heart. Hence, the decline in muscle mass has serious implications for the functioning of the body as a whole.

Despite the unforeseeable circumstances that come with aging, some lifestyle choices may add to the preexisting complications that come with the loss of muscle mass. A poor diet that lacks important nutrients and proteins essential for building muscles can weaken the process of muscle protein synthesis, which is essential for building both cellular and physiological structures in the body. Furthermore, lack of exercise or physical activity creates a wasting away of the muscles due to disuse. When there is a decreased use of the muscles, the body interprets this as them no longer being needed; hence, less energy is used to maintain them, leading to them being reduced in size and strength. To prevent this from occurring, it is important to engage in physical activity, especially exercises that involve resistance, such as strength training (Volpi et al., 2004).

BONE HEALTH

In addition to the loss of muscle mass, another crucial aspect impacted by age is bone health. The bone structure is essential for enabling movement and supporting vital organs such as the brain and heart, among many others. Any deterioration in the quality of the bone structure, whether in size or volume, can not only affect mobility but could cause or exacerbate injuries, weakening one's strength to do activities that, under different circumstances, would normally be seen as simple and safe.

In women, hormonal imbalances, such as a reduction in the estrogen hormone that occurs during menopause, can affect the natural process of bone renewal or formation. Therefore, bone density, measured by bone resistance and mineral constituents within bone tissues, declines with age. This condition is named osteoporosis, which is recognizable not only by a decline in bone density but also by the deterioration of the bone structure. Consequently, this results in frail bones that can be easily fractured.

Although osteoporosis is often age-related, certain lifestyle choices can intensify its impact, such as a nutrient-deficient diet, drug and alcohol use, and a lack of exercise. Nutrients such as vitamin D and calcium are essential for bone health. Vitamin D aids bone health by absorbing calcium, giving strength and structure to the bone. Therefore, having the correct diet is important.

In spite of the fact that a proper diet can aid bone health, destructive behaviors such as excessive drinking and smoking can counter any effort toward improving bone health. Heavy smoking allows the nicotine substance in cigarettes to infiltrate the body, slowing down the process of bone formation by disturbing the absorption of calcium into the bone. As a result, the bones lack the necessary minerals to avoid frailty. Similarly, heavy drinking increases hormones such as cortisol and parathyroid, which lead to bone impairment by draining the calcium from bones.

Apart from eating healthy and limiting smoking and drinking habits, exercise also plays a role in bone formation and structure. Bone tissues can be strengthened through regular exercise, increasing the density of the bone and remodeling its structure, restoring it to good condition. Therefore, a well-rounded lifestyle is important for bone health to avoid any risk of bone fractures due to the wearing down of bone tissues. Lastly, impaired bones affect the body's strength to do daily activities, limiting mobility and function due to the risk of injury with each force exerted to perform a particular activity.

As mentioned above, multiple factors connected to aging have a negative impact on muscle mass and bone density, which in turn affect the overall strength of the body to move and function normally. However, as observed, many of these factors can be actively mitigated through a healthy lifestyle that includes a nutritious diet and regular exercise (Volpi et al., 2004).

2. Addressing Common Misconceptions About Strength Training in Older Adults

Although strength training is known to have many benefits across all age groups, common misconceptions about strength training may prevent people from incorporating it into their exercise routine, fearing that it may be more detrimental than beneficial.

Let us look at some common misconceptions about strength training for older adults and disprove them.

Strength Training Is Only for Younger People

This thought process comes from the impression that once you reach a certain age, you cannot take part in certain activities as you are more prone to injuries. The main concern in this statement might come from the illusion that there is a certain period in life when it is safe to pursue building or strengthening one's muscles: in one's youth. Anything past this period is seen as dangerous and unadvisable. On social media, strength training is often painted as an activity for youth or professional athletes, which spreads a narrative that you have to be young and fit to pursue strength training.

Contrary to popular belief, you do not need to be young or fit to partake in strength training. It is actually exceptionally important that people of all ages take part in strength training because of the benefits that are imperative as we grow older. As with most things, it is important to be informed, guaranteeing that you have the correct posture, tools, and movements to ensure safe practice (Seguin et al., 2003).

OLDER PEOPLE ARE PRONE TO INJURY FROM STRENGTH TRAINING

Similarly to the misconception of youth being best fit for strength training, many may fear that strength training may cause further harm to those already faced with age-related illnesses. The belief is that strength training is too strenuous and challenging for older people and may cause muscle injuries or joint pains or even aggravate existing health conditions.

However, as mentioned previously, strength training is suitable for all age groups and can be adjusted to one's individual needs. Hence, it is important to seek advice from one's doctor or physician about the extent to which one can incorporate strength training into their exercise routine (Seguin et al., 2003).

LIFTING WEIGHTS MAKES WOMEN BULKY

Many women avoid strength training, afraid of the aesthetic changes because they don't want to look bulky like men tend to do. Strength training tends to help tone muscles, improve metabolism, and enhance overall strength. The truth, however, is that women do not produce enough testosterone to gain excessive muscle mass from strength training (*What Women Need to Know*, n.d.).

Cardiovascular Exercises Are Sufficient

This is one of the biggest misconceptions in the fitness realm: the assumption that doing cardio workouts, like walking briskly, swimming, or cycling, a few times a week is a sufficient amount of exercise. While doing cardio on its own is important for your heart and overall health, it is not enough. Strength training is necessary to address muscle strength and bone density; this only becomes more important as you age, not less. Strength training is necessary for better mobility and reduced risk of falling (Volpi et al., 2004).

It Is Too Late to Start Strength Training

Some might think that they are too old or weak to start strength training, that their window of opportunity has already passed. This is not true since people in their '80s and '90s can benefit from strength training. Adaptions to movements can be made, amount of repetitions completed can be adjusted, and the equipment needed can be changed depending on the fitness levels and ability of the person.

This book will show a few different adaptions to some strength training exercises; however, it is also important to talk to your health practitioner and maybe rope in the help of a professional trainer (Seguin et al., 2003).

The point is that it is not only possible but important to incorporate strength training into our lives.

STRENGTH TRAINING REQUIRES A GYM MEMBERSHIP OR EXPENSIVE EQUIPMENT

While some prefer to join a gym and use its facilities—including the trainer—others might prefer using household items. Look over the suggestions in the book, ask for suggestions from others or online, and think outside the box. Many roads lead to Rome!

EXPERIENCING PAIN AND DISCOMFORT DURING AND AFTER STRENGTH TRAINING IS NORMAL

There is a large difference between muscle soreness from exercising and significant pain and persistent discomfort. Hence, it is important, never mind your age, to slowly move into a workout routine. It is impossible to start running and think you will be able to accomplish an entire marathon immediately. Try out a variety of exercises and take note of the level of comfort that you feel. Work your way up to more repetitions and a wider variety of movements as your body becomes stronger and more accustomed to the exercises (*Pain and Injuries*, n.d.).

It is important to remember the following while exercising: Do not move too quickly, and stop the moment you feel any sharp pain. Incorporating exercise into your lifestyle is a journey; be patient and listen to your body. Misinterpreting significant pain for muscle soreness could cause discouragement, and you ultimately end up giving up on strength training completely.

ONLY HEAVY WEIGHTS ARE EFFECTIVE

The efficacy and sustainability of strength training lie in progressive overload. This is when you start off with a manageable amount of movement and slowly increase the number of repetitions and types of movements as time progresses, and you feel able to do more (Heimlich, 2024).

If you start with an amount that pushes you past your comfort and leaves you feeling drained and in significant pain and discomfort, it is not sustainable or good for your body.

SUMMARY

It is evident from the arguments made above that a lack of knowledge and exposure to the true benefits of strength training may cause older adults to shy away from engaging in strength training. However, this does not have to be the case, and that is what this book seeks to achieve.

3. Overcoming Barriers and Fears Associated With Strength Training

Hand in hand with common misconceptions regarding strength training, multiple other barriers stop many from starting their strength training journey. We will shortly discuss these barriers as well as a few suggestions on how to work past them.

Psychological Barriers

Psychological barriers refer to the fear of getting injured during exercise, worrying about being judged by others, feeling embarrassed, or simply lacking the confidence needed to participate in strength training activities.

For many, the fear of injury and the lack of confidence are interconnected issues. When an individual doubts their ability to perform an exercise correctly, they may avoid attempting it altogether out of fear of potential harm. This cycle of insecurity can prevent them from taking the necessary steps to improve their physical well-being, choosing to stop after only attempting an exercise once. As they grow older, they are more prone to serious injury and thus fear getting hurt exercising. With this in mind, it is important to remember that it is impossible to avoid ever getting hurt, and strength training reduces the severity and likelihood of injury (Volpi et al., 2004).

Some people tend to get anxious when exercising because they worry about others watching them. It can feel overwhelming when you are trying to focus on figuring out how to complete an exercise right, but you get distracted because you feel like others are observing you attentively. This is especially the case when you age and feel like you are not as capable as you once were. Doubts fill your mind: *Is my form correct? Did I do that move correctly? Am I too big, too old, or too lost to be here lifting weights?*

The reality is that everyone starts somewhere. It is rare for someone to begin a new activity and be good at it right away. It's important to remember that everyone has been a beginner at some point. Even the most seasoned *gymgoers* started with the basics and progressed over time. The key is to focus on your own journey without comparing yourself to others.

Nobody becomes an expert overnight. It's completely normal to feel uncertain when trying something new, especially in a gym setting. Take your time working through the exercises in this book, look at tutorials available on the Internet, and remember that practice makes perfect!

Embrace the learning process and be patient with yourself. Each workout is an opportunity to improve and grow, regardless of what others may or may not be thinking. To ease the fear of judgment, try to tune out external distractions. Focus on your workout routine, breathing, and form. Listen to music or your favorite comfort series in the background, and try not to let your mind wander. Remember that most people at the gym are focused on their own workouts and do not pay close attention to others.

Keep in mind that everyone's fitness journey is unique. It's essential to honor your progress, setbacks, and achievements without comparing yourself to others. Embrace the challenges and victories along the way, and focus on your personal growth and well-being. By staying committed to your fitness goals and prioritizing self-care, you can overcome the fear of judgment and enjoy a fulfilling gym experience.

PHYSICAL BARRIERS

Many fear that they are not fit or able enough to start strength training. *What if the lightest weight is too heavy? What if I cannot complete a movement? It might just feel easier to avoid it altogether.*

Additionally, starting a new form of exercise that the body is not used to will cause initial soreness and discomfort, which deters many from continuing, as they either do not like the feeling or fear that they have injured themselves.

On the other hand, many people have some type of health condition or mobility issue that deters them from completing certain exercises as is. It is exceptionally important to keep your conditions and the accompanying restrictions in mind and to check with your healthcare practitioner whether you can safely attempt the exercises. They will be able to inform you if it is something that you are more than welcome to try or which exercises you should avoid.

It is important to remember that completing an activity in the manners shown in this book is not the beginning and the end; modified variations are available for most exercises, and many times, you can do a safer, similar exercise instead of a more complex one. You are also able to exchange the weights with a resistance band, which lowers the impact. Besides, it is completely fine to first practice moving into the movement until it feels comfortable and you feel ready to add weights.

Do not give up on strength training due to physical limitations. If something does not work for you, do a bit of research, ask someone with more knowledge, and be open to failing, trying again, and trying something else!

LOGISTICAL BARRIERS

Juggling work, school, and social commitments leaves little time for activities like strength training in most people's hectic schedules. It is important to specifically put time aside for personal care, which includes looking after your health, in other words, exercising. Exercising must not be seen as a chore; rather, it is a major aspect of your life. Many people do not have easy access to the correct hardware for strength training like weights, and acquiring these items or a gym membership might not be financially possible right now.

If this is the case for you, please do not give up! There are so many different, more affordable, and accessible options. All it takes is a bit of research and creative thinking! Home workouts are an option, as well as making weights out of water bottles, using a resistance band, or saving to buy a single pair of cost-effective hand weights. There are many different options to start strength training in a way that your pocket feels comfortable.

It is also important to note that while multiple strength training exercises require equipment, many do not. You have the freedom to add and remove exercises from your workout routine as you try them out and decide what you feel most comfortable with.

Social and Cultural Barriers

Older adults might not have a supportive social network due to misconceptions about strength training and their physical abilities as they age. Strength training is not only beneficial to people of all ages but also exceptionally important for their overall health (Volpi et al., 2004). Thus, it is important to raise awareness about these misconceptions with friends and family members. It is also vital to not let others' opinions bother you. It is your body and your health on the line.

Having a group of supportive peers is a great alternative; find a group of people online or join an in-person class. Having others' support around you makes the world's difference.

At the end of the day, if you stick to your workout program, you will show everyone that did not believe in you wrong.

Educational Barriers

Lack of knowledge about strength training is one of the main reasons that people avoid it completely. This is where this book comes in. It not only discusses the urgent importance of adding strength training to your daily life, but it also explains how to go about starting this new journey. A variety of exercise movements are available, as well as ways to set up your own workout program and essential nutritious facts that must be kept in mind during your strength training prepping.

Not understanding how to complete an exercise in a way you are comfortable with tends to make you avoid trying it. Various sources are available online with visual examples of how the movements must be completed, as well as possible adaptations that can be implemented. If an exercise is too difficult, could it be adjusted by trading the weights for a resistance band? Or is there an alternative movement that can be done to reduce the amount of pressure on a certain area? You will be able to find that out by reading this book, talking to others who also do strength training, asking a trainer, or searching on the Internet!

It is important to remember that few people start off without any hiccups. For the large part, it is a learning process, one that you should not be afraid to embark upon.

SUMMARY

Many different barriers and fears might make us second-guess our strength training journey, but it is important not to shy away from what we fear. Rather, we must seek to understand the core of the problems and resolve them.

Strength training is not something that can be exchanged for a different type of exercise, and its importance thereof cannot be stated enough.

Remember: You can do difficult things!

4. BENEFITS OF STRENGTH TRAINING FOR OLDER WOMEN

Aging does not have to turn into an undesirable or unwanted stage in life that one wishes to avoid. It may sound too good to be true, but even as we mature, we can still retain the things we admire about being young to a large extent.

The number of years added to our lives should never determine the level of enthusiasm, passion, and energy needed to cultivate the lives we desire. Nevertheless, we cannot naively assume that this is easily attainable without a plan or a guided way of living that can enhance its possibility. The intent of this book is to provide a clear and easy-to-follow guideline on how to feel stronger, rejuvenated, and more flexible as mature women through strength training.

Numerous benefits can be gained from strength training, but let us begin with the one benefit implied by the term itself: strength. As mentioned before, strength is a phenomenon that becomes increasingly elusive with age due to the loss of muscle mass over time. The good news, however, is that muscle mass is not irrecoverable. Our bodies have the incredible ability to adapt to different pressures when consistently exposed to them. The same applies to strength training. The more strain we put on our bodies, the more they learn to resist it. With weight lifting or resistance training, stress is placed on the muscles, causing slight damage to the muscle fibers. The body then responds by repairing the muscles and building new muscle tissue to prepare the body to withstand any pressure of that nature in the future. With continued exposure to strength training, the communication pattern between the brain and the muscles becomes more efficient. This results in less neural energy required to recruit for muscle building (Volpi et al., 2004). Hence, one not only grows in strength but also in endurance, even when undertaking hefty activities.

Strength training not only strengthens us physically but also mentally. It enhances cognitive function and reduces the risk of cognitive decline. Moreover, it helps increase blood flow to the brain and stimulates the growth of new brain cells. As we age, a decline in memory and cognitive function takes place, but strength training can curb this (Volpi et al., 2004).

In addition to the strength built from the process of muscle repair, strength training aids in maintaining bone density. As previously stated, various age-related factors contribute to the decline in bone health. Strength training counters the negative impact of these factors by inflicting mechanical stress on the bones and, therefore, stimulating the process of bone formation. During weight lifting or resistance training, stress is placed on the muscles and transferred to the bones, prompting osteoblast activity in which new bone cells are formed in response to the physical strain placed on the bones. New tissue is then formed, replacing the old and damaged bone tissue; this is called bone remodeling. As a result, bone density is improved, giving the body structure and increasing its ability to withstand pressure (Volpi et al., 2004).

Another way in which strength training exercises help with body structure is by activating the different muscle groups, stimulating movement, aiding in joint flexibility, promoting appropriate body posture, and facilitating coordinated motion. For instance, strength training exercises that engage core muscles, such as squats, contribute to building a strong core, which provides stability to the spine and pelvis, training the body to maintain good posture, thereby reducing the likelihood of lower back pain or muscle strain. As various muscle groups are activated, the muscles around the joints become more stable, preventing joint stiffness and enhancing flexibility and balance. Furthermore, strength training enhances the communication between the brain and muscles, allowing for more controlled movements that maintain stability and improve balance. Consequently, good posture, balance, and flexibility provide the body with additional support and help prevent the risks of falls or injuries (Bielecki & Tadi, 2021).

In light of the benefits of strength training toward building muscle mass, increasing bone density, improving balance and flexibility, and enhancing overall strength, it is not surprising that strength training can assist in slowing down the progression of chronic illnesses such as arthritis and osteoporosis. In this setting, strength training results in extra support of the bone structure, providing the body with a sense of balance and coordination, which, in turn, reduces the risk of falling and causing further harm to existing fractures (Volpi et al., 2004).

Furthermore, symptoms of chronic illnesses, such as joint pain and stiffness, are relieved through the activation of muscles during strength training, leaving us feeling less hindered by the challenges that come with aging. This, in turn, has a positive impact on our mental health, as the less trapped we feel in our bodies, the healthier we feel, and the better decisions we are able to make for ourselves (Volpi et al., 2004).

The benefits of strength training are numerous, and they provide us with independence for a longer amount of time, so we require less assistance or only need assistance at a later stage in our lives.

Considering the benefits mentioned thus far, strength training contributes as a source of energy and vitality, allowing the body and mind, regardless of age, to have a sense of autonomy to perform day-to-day activities with more ease than expected.

5. Assessing Current Fitness Level

S trength training is a gratifying pursuit that can elevate your overall physical fitness and well-being. To successfully embark on this journey, it is vital to possess a clear understanding of your current fitness level. Incorporating strength training into your routine is indispensable, but equally essential is comprehending your body's dynamics and physical capacities to prevent injuries or exacerbating existing conditions.

Accurately tracking changes in your body weight, measurements, and body fat percentage monitors progress and serves as a powerful motivational tool. Establish a solid foundation for your strength training journey by progressing steadily, listening to your body, and staying dedicated to your fitness goals. Consistency and commitment are key to long-term success in your pursuit of strength and health.

Furthermore, stay vigilant for warning signs as you delve into your new exercise regimen. Consult your healthcare provider to educate yourself on important red flags like dizziness, shortness of breath, or chest pain, which could indicate underlying issues.

Recognizing these warning signs acts as a safety precaution during your workouts. If you encounter any of these symptoms, seek guidance from your doctor on the necessary steps, whether they involve taking a break, seeking medical assistance, or adjusting your routine.

TIP

Have a small book or online document where you write down the information about your fitness level before starting a workout. This is a wonderful tool to track how you have progressed along your journey.

Let's walk through the steps to help you kick-start your strength training venture.

CONSULTING WITH YOUR HEALTH CARE PROVIDER

It's important to talk to your health care provider before starting any new workout plan, especially if you have existing health issues. Your doctor knows your medical history and can give you tips; they can tell you which exercises are safe and which to avoid, taking your unique health circumstances into consideration. They could also inform you of any warning signs that you must be on the lookout for; for example, if you feel a sharp pain in your chest, stop the exercise immediately and call your doctor.

They might give you the green light to start but possibly suggest modifications to certain movements to keep you safe. Your doctor's guidance can make your workout sessions more effective and enjoyable. Remember, your health comes first, so don't hesitate to ask for advice at any point in your fitness journey.

Completing Self-Assessments of Your Physical Condition

Consider your general health status, recent injuries, or surgeries that may affect your training. Testing your mobility, flexibility, endurance, and strength gives you a baseline from which to work, providing you with an idea as to what you are able to do and a clearer picture of what you wish to work toward.

As these are only baseline tests and your body might not be used to the movements, remember to move slowly and listen to your body. Do not force yourself into a position that creates much discomfort for you, as this might lead to injury.

Please note that the following are only a few of the many ways you can test your mobility, flexibility, endurance, and strength.

Mobility Tests

The way you move your body reveals a lot about your physical health. Completing a mobility test will also give you a clear indicator in regards to what exercises you will be able to complete and whether adaptations might be necessary for certain exercises (Howe, 2019). It is important to note that there are many different types of mobility tests, and these are only a few examples; if you struggle to complete one of them, feel more than welcome to look for other examples on the Internet!

Shoulder Mobility Test

Gently reach one hand over your shoulder and down your back while the other hand goes up your back from the waist. The aim is to touch your fingertips together. This simple test helps you understand how well your shoulders can move and their range of motion.

Elbow Flexion and Extension Test

Assume a comfortable position, either standing or sitting, with your arms relaxed at your sides. Lift one arm in front of you, bend your elbow, and bring your palm toward your shoulder, attempting to touch your shoulder with your fingertips. Take notice of the range of motion and any discomfort or restrictions. Next, extend the same arm straight out in front of you, fully straightening your elbow to align your arm with your shoulder. Pay attention to the range of motion and any discomfort or restrictions. Adequate ability to touch your shoulder and fully extend your arm signifies good elbow mobility. Difficulty touching your shoulder, inability to fully extend your arm, or experiencing pain may indicate restricted elbow mobility, stiffness, or an underlying issue that requires attention.

Enhance elbow flexibility with targeted stretches for the biceps, triceps, and forearms. Integrate exercises like bicep curls, triceps extensions, and wrist flexor stretches to bolster elbow strength in your workout regimen.

Wrist Mobility Test–Prayer Stretch Test

Sit or stand comfortably. Place your palms together in front of your chest, fingers pointing upward, and forearms parallel to the ground. Slowly lower your hands while keeping your palms pressed together until you feel a mild stretch in your wrists and forearms. Ensure your palms are together and your forearms are parallel throughout. Hold for a few seconds to assess motion range, discomfort, or restrictions. The goal is to lower your hands to a 90° angle without discomfort. Beyond this angle indicates good wrist mobility, while difficulty or pain may suggest limited mobility or tightness. To enhance flexibility, include wrist flexor and extensor stretches. Strengthen with exercises like wrist curls, reverse wrist curls, and grip strengthening in your routine.

Knee-To-Wall Test

Stand in front of a wall with your toes a couple of inches from it. Place your hands on the wall for support. Bend one knee toward the wall, ensuring your heel stays on the ground. Adjust the distance between your toes and the wall until you find the farthest point where your knee can touch the wall without raising your heel. Measure the distance from your big toe to the wall using a ruler or tape measure. Repeat the process with the opposite knee and compare the results. Ideally, both knees should touch the wall with your toes positioned 4–5 in.—10–12 cm—away from it without lifting your heels. Noticeable differences between the 2 sides might suggest mobility issues that could be improved by specific stretch and strength exercises such as leg extensions, hamstring curls, and calf raises. It is advisable to consult a physical therapist or healthcare professional before commencing any new exercise regimen.

Ankle Mobility Test

Kneel on one knee with the other foot flat on the ground in front of you. See if you can lean forward enough to move your knee past your toes without lifting your heel. This movement can show how flexible your ankles are.

Thoracic Spine Mobility Test

Find a comfortable spot on the floor, cross your legs, and place a broomstick across your shoulders. Slowly rotate your torso to the left and right without moving your hips. This test helps understand your thoracic spine mobility.

Hip Mobility Test–Thomas Test

To start, find a sturdy, even surface like a bed or treatment table. Sit at the edge with your legs hanging down, then lie down and bring one knee toward your chest, holding it securely with both hands. Ensure your lower back remains flat against the surface, avoiding any arching. Check how the hanging leg is positioned. If it stays level with the knee bent at 90°, it indicates good hip flexor mobility. Keep an eye on the hanging thigh. If it rises or the knee straightens, it signals tightness in the hip flexors. Repeat the same on the other side to assess hip flexibility. Confirm that the hanging leg's thigh lies flat on the surface, with the knee bent close to 90°. Thigh lifting hints at tightness in the iliopsoas muscle, a crucial hip flexor. A knee extension suggests tightness in the rectus femoris, part of the quadriceps group and a hip flexor.

For a hip flexor stretch, kneel on one knee while sliding the other foot forward. Slowly push your hips forward, ensuring an upright torso. To perform a quadriceps stretch, stand on one leg and draw the other foot toward your buttocks. During glute bridges, lay on your back with your knees bent and feet flat on the ground, then lift your hips by activating your glute muscles. Engage in lunges by stepping forward into a lunge position, keeping the back leg straight to stretch the hip flexors while building lower-body strength.

Flexibility Check

Flexibility is crucial for optimal body movement and overall health. Practicing your mobility is important to ensure you do not injure yourself when moving into strength training exercises. If you are not very flexible, it is completely fine! It just means that you need to be careful and move slowly into strength training exercises and, above all else, listen to your body. If the movement feels very uncomfortable or you feel a sharp pain, stop immediately (Parker, 2019).

When you perform flexibility checks, it's essential to listen to your body and avoid pushing yourself to the point of extreme discomfort or injury risk.

- **To assess hamstring and lower back flexibility:** Sit on the floor with your legs extended. Reach forward without bending your knees. See how close you are to reaching your toes. Once again, do not push yourself to the point of severe discomfort as this will not provide accurate results and could lead to injury.
- **To assess trunk flexibility:** Lie prone and raise your upper body as high as you can while maintaining your hips in contact with the ground to assess lower back flexibility. It is advisable to perform this action on a firm surface, as a soft mattress may cause sinking or discomfort and yield negligible outcomes.
- **To assess quadriceps flexibility:** For insights into quadriceps flexibility, stand on one leg and lift your foot toward your buttocks, aiming to bring your heel close to your glutes. This action assesses quadriceps flexibility effectively.

Endurance Evaluation

Testing your endurance when planning to add a strength training program might sound off, but there is validity to this evaluation. Strength training largely focuses on building muscle mass, power, and strength, but it is important to have a certain level of muscular and cardiovascular endurance to enhance your strength training performance and overall fitness. Better cardiovascular and muscular endurance can reduce the time needed to recover between sets, which allows for more efficient and intense workouts.

The Six-Minute Walk Test

Ensure you are walking on a flat surface, wear comfortable attire, and have a stopwatch or timer in hand. Measure the distance from one end of a room to another. Once you have warmed up by stretching a bit or walking up and down a bit, it is time to start your laps. Start walking up and down the room until the end of the 6-minute mark, remembering the amount of laps you made. Multiply the number of laps by the distance in the room we mentioned beforehand; for example, 15 laps on a 20-m path amounts to 300 m. Write this down as well as anything else that you experienced, like breathlessness or dizziness. The average for a woman over 60 is approximately 500–650 m, but it can differ depending on other health conditions and fitness levels (*Six Minute Walk Test*, n.d.).

Strength Assessment

There are many different ways that you can test your strength; below are two simple tests that will examine your lower- and upper-body strength. Regularly performing these tests can help track improvements and maintain functional power for daily activities. If any exercise causes pain, stop immediately and consult a health care professional (*Senior Citizen Fitness Test*, n.d.).

To Assess Lower-Body Strength: Chair Stand Test

You will require a sturdy chair without armrests and a stopwatch.

Place the chair against a wall to prevent it from moving. Sit in the middle of the chair with your feet flat on the floor, shoulder-width apart. Cross your arms over your chest. Stand up fully, then sit back down. This counts as 1 repetition. Repeat as many times as possible in 30 seconds. Count the number of times you can stand up and sit down in 30 seconds. The average amount of repetitions for someone in their early '60s is 12–17 reps, and 9–13 reps for someone in their early '80s.

To Assess Upper-Body strength: Arm Curl Test

You will require a 5-lb dumbbell (2.3 kg), a chair with armrests, and a stopwatch.

Sit on the chair with your back straight and feet flat on the floor. Hold the dumbbell in your dominant hand with your arm extended down by your side. Curl the dumbbell by bending your elbow and bringing your hand toward your shoulder. Lower the dumbbell back to the starting position. This counts as 1 repetition. Repeat as many times as possible in 30 seconds. Count the number of arm curls completed in 30 seconds. The average amount of repetitions for someone in their early '60s is 15–20 reps, and 11–16 reps for someone in their early '80s.

Balance Examination

Maintaining balance is vital for steadiness and synchronization. It plays a crucial role in your overall well-being, as well as the security and effectiveness of workout routines. Balance is essential for minimizing the risk of falling and injuring yourself. Furthermore, it boosts your ability to execute exercises accurately, thereby improving your overall performance and satisfaction. Ensuring balance also safeguards and bolsters joint health; during strength training, proper balance distributes weight and pressure evenly across your joints, lessening the chances of injury, deterioration, and strain.

It is important to test your balance before you start strength training exercises to ensure that the type of exercises that you do cater to your balance abilities (Berg-Hansen et al., 2023). Here are two balance tests:

1. **Single-leg stand test:** This test helps you assess your balance and body awareness. It is best to have something supportive, like a chair or couch, close by to stabilize yourself if you lose your balance and stumble. Stand on one leg with your eyes open for as long as you can, and then repeat with your eyes closed. Repeat for the other leg.

2. **The Y balance test:** Stand on one leg and reach the other leg out in three different directions to assess your overall balance. Start off by lightly lifting your leg out in front of you. Record how long you are able to hold the pose before you start losing your balance. Next, lightly lift your leg to the side, assessing once again how long you are able to hold the pose. Lastly, lightly lift your left backward. You do not have to lift your leg too far; the point is to test your balance, not injure yourself or test your flexibility.

Commence strength training exercises very cautiously if your balance is not optimal; improving balance is vital to minimize injury risks, but you can still start strength training even if your balance is not the best. Your workout routine should include specific balance exercises such as single-leg stands, heel-to-toe walks, and balance board activities. Consistent practice is essential for enhancing and preserving balance. Hence, strive to include balance exercises in your routine multiple times weekly.

BODY COMPOSITION ANALYSIS

Body composition analysis is "a methodology utilized to ascertain the proportions of distinct components constituting an individual's body weight, such as fat, muscle, bone, and water." Unlike mere weight measurement or body mass index (BMI), body composition analysis offers a comprehensive understanding of a person's physical condition and overall health status.

A body composition analysis, like the BMI test, can be relatively costly, prompting many individuals who exercise for fitness to rather just consult their health care provider for recommendations. While these tests yield valuable information, they are not obligatory before commencing strength training (Duren et al., 2008).

Body composition analysis encompasses the following components and their significance:

- Body fat

  o Essential fat: Vital for normal physiological functions and located in various organs and tissues.
  o Storage fat: Accumulates in adipose tissue, either subcutaneously or around internal organs.

- Muscle mass: Essential for movement, strength, and metabolism.
- Bone density: Crucial for structural support and mobility.
- Body water: Critical for physiological processes like digestion and temperature regulation.

Various methods are employed for body composition analysis:

- *BIA devices:* Estimates body composition by measuring body fat percentage and lean muscle mass through the use of a harmless electrical current. These devices analyze the resistance encountered by the current as it passes through the body, with muscle and water offering less resistance compared to fat. There are different types of BIA devices available: handheld devices for upper-body measurements, scale-based devices for lower-body measurements, and multi-frequency segmental devices for detailed assessments of specific body segments. These devices are affordable and simple to use at home, with measurements being quick and noninvasive. However, the accuracy of BIA results can be influenced by factors such as hydration levels and recent physical activity. Regular calibration and adherence to testing conditions are key for reliable measurements. BIA is valuable for monitoring body composition changes, tailoring fitness and nutrition plans, and assessing the effectiveness of lifestyle changes for long-term health management.

- *Dual-energy X-ray absorptiometry (DEXA):* It is a highly accurate method using low-dose X-rays. The individual lies on a table while a scanning arm passes over the body, taking about 10–20 minutes for the scan. The 2 X-ray beams pass through the body and are absorbed by different bodily tissues at different rates. Fat, muscle, and bone each absorb X-rays differently. By analyzing differences in absorption rates, DEXA provides detailed imaging and analysis of body composition, offering precise measurements of bone density, body fat percentage, and lean muscle mass. Renowned for its accuracy, DEXA is considered one of the most precise methods for body composition analysis.

- *Skinfold calipers:* Utilized to measure skinfold thickness and estimate the individual's total body fat percentage. These affordable tools gauge subcutaneous fat thickness at designated body sites, including the triceps, biceps, subscapular, and suprailiac regions. Achieving precision demands proficient skills and consistency in measurement techniques, emphasizing the importance of professional training or mastering the correct methodology for dependable outcomes. To ensure accuracy in tracking, consistent measurements at identical sites under similar conditions are imperative. Although effective for approximating body fat levels, skinfold measurements may be slightly less precise compared to sophisticated methods such as DEXA scans. The technique involves grasping and raising the skinfold away from the underlying muscle for calipers to determine thickness in millimeters. Integration of measurements from multiple sites into equations or charts aids in estimating the overall body fat percentage.

- *Hydrostatic weighing: Hydrostatic weighing,* also known as *underwater weighing,* is "a precise method used to measure body density and fat percentage by weighing a person underwater." This technique is grounded in Archimedes' principle, which equates the buoyant force on a submerged object to the weight of the displaced fluid. Initially, the individual is weighed on land before being immersed in a water tank for a subsequent weighing. The discrepancy between these two weights is utilized to ascertain body density. By leveraging the principle that fat tissue is less dense than water while muscle tissue is denser, the body density calculation approximates the ratio of fat to lean mass. Regarded as a gold standard for body composition assessment, hydrostatic weighing provides consistent and accurate measurements when executed properly. However, its reliance on specialized equipment and facilities renders it costlier and less accessible than alternative methods. In addition, some individuals may find the process uncomfortable due to the need to submerge in water and exhale fully to gauge residual lung volume. Compared to other techniques, hydrostatic weighing is time-consuming and involves several steps for precise outcomes.

The Significance of Body Composition Analysis

It offers a comprehensive health overview beyond weight or BMI. Additionally, it provides you with an in-depth understanding of your overall health and thus helps you design your workout according to your needs, as well as a suggested nutrition program to support the areas most needed (e.g., what to eat to help with low bone density). Monitoring your body composition will give you insights into how your training regime changes your body, lowering your storage fat, increasing muscle mass and muscle density, etc. It can also identify unhealthy body fat levels linked to chronic diseases.

In conclusion, body composition analysis is a valuable tool for comprehending the components contributing to body weight and health. By providing detailed insights into fat, muscle, bone, and water levels, it aids individuals and professionals in making informed decisions regarding fitness, nutrition, and health strategies. Whether for enhancing athletic performance, health monitoring, or customizing fitness programs, body composition analysis offers a comprehensive assessment superior to traditional methods like weighing yourself on a scale and completing a BMI test (Duren et al., 2008).

6. SETTING REALISTIC GOALS AND DESIGNING AN EFFECTIVE WORKOUT PROGRAM

Embarking on a strength training journey at 60 years old is a praiseworthy choice that can greatly improve health, vitality, and overall well-being. To succeed in the long run, it's crucial to establish achievable goals.

At this point, you have already conducted a comprehensive evaluation of your current fitness level, covering body composition, flexibility, strength, and cardiovascular fitness. If you decide to seek advice from a trainer or your healthcare provider, you have that information to guide your decisions as well. Now comes the fun. However, sometimes, the time-consuming process of setting goals and designing strength training recommends seeking guidance from a fitness expert. Hence, seek medical approval and discuss with your health care provider to ascertain any health issues or physical constraints that should influence your workout plan.

SETTING REALISTIC GOALS

Define Your Objectives

This step is exceptionally important to set your objectives because this is what will drive you to continue through the more difficult days. Establish short-term goals for the next few weeks and long-term objectives for the upcoming months and the first year. Clear goals help you stay focused and motivated throughout your fitness journey. Looking back at your journal, seeing and hearing how you have improved is exceptional motivation. The first key step to consider before engaging in any strength training workout is what you aim to achieve from it.

As individuals, we have different reasons to see the importance of implementing an exercise routine in our lives, specifically one that incorporates strength training. These reasons can range from having the desire to look better and feel better, managing and improving specific health conditions, increasing physical strength and endurance, being more flexible, and–or obtaining more balance. Whatever the reason is, that is the *why* that can keep one going, and hence, it needs to be personal to each individual.

However, in assessing our fitness goals, it is important to be aware of factors that could potentially restrict the body from engaging in certain exercises. These include but are not limited to, medical conditions such as arthritis or heart disease, a short-term illness, pregnancy, physical injuries, fractures, and–or persistent pain or discomfort in certain parts of the body. If one has any physical or medical constraints, these need to be noted as they will determine the type, level, and intensity of the exercises that they can engage in.

Make Your Goals SMART

Setting *specific, measurable, achievable, relevant, and time-bound* goals is key to transforming your aspirations into tangible accomplishments.

Specify your objectives clearly. Instead of a vague goal like, "I want to get stronger," define it as: "I aim to lift a 10-lb weight in a 4-month period."

Ensure that your progress is *measurable.* For example, set targets such as reducing body fat by 5% or completing 15 squats in a day with proper form.

Guarantee your goals are *achievable* and within reach based on your current fitness level and available resources. Gradual advancement is essential for success. It is not fair to yourself to say, "I aim to complete 50 squats per day in a week," when you are unable to complete a single squat today. It will be demotivating if you are unable to achieve this.

Make sure your goals are *relevant* to your overall health and fitness objectives—choose aims that are meaningful and impactful to you. If you have a leg injury, it is best to work on upper-body strength training until the leg is healed. If your goal is aimed at strengthening your legs, you will feel frustrated as it is not something you are able to do.

Establish a clear *time frame* for achieving your goals. Setting short-term objectives, such as accomplishing a goal within three months, can help maintain your motivation. Moreover, setting long-term goals will remind you of the bigger picture and the reason for keeping strong.

Designing an Effective Workout Program

Selecting Suitable Exercises

When choosing exercises, focus on ones that target different muscle groups and support daily movements. Make sure the exercises align with your fitness level and any medical conditions you may have. Remember, if any exercise creates severe discomfort or hurts, avoid it, at least until a later stage, when you have progressed in your strength training journey. Having a variety of exercises that you interchange on your exercise days prevents boredom and ensures a well-rounded workout routine. For example, on one day, do a combination of two upper-body exercises and two lower-body exercises, and the next day you exercise, do two core and two different lower-body exercises, etc.

Planning Your Workout Routine

Plan your weekly workout schedule by determining the frequency of strength training sessions; typically, 2–3 times a week helps maintain muscle mass, which supports metabolism and bone health. Remember to rest between sessions to avoid overtraining. Start each session with a 5–10 minute warm-up to prime your body, then proceed to targeted exercises such as those for legs, back, and core. Keep your workout sessions between 30 and 60 minutes, warming up and cooling down included. Shorter sessions are good if you are just starting out but gradually increase as you get fitter.

Repetitions indicate "how many times you consecutively perform a specific exercise movement," while sets denote "a series of repetitions done without interruption." For example, if you finish 10 reps of a bicep curl before resting, that counts as 1 set of 10 reps. If your workout plan specifies 3 sets of 10 reps for a particular exercise, you'll complete 10 reps, take a break, do another 10 reps, rest once more, and finish with a final set of 10 reps. Start with easy exercises and work your way up. Use weights or resistance bands to make exercises harder gradually. Besides, when doing cardio, make sure it's moderate to keep your heart healthy without overdoing it.

When determining the number of repetitions and sets, ensure it's a manageable quantity that you can gradually escalate as your strength progresses. Incorporate a 5–10 minute cooldown at the end of your session to aid muscle recovery and alleviate stiffness.

Progressive Overload

Progressive overload is "when you slowly make exercises harder to keep challenging your muscles." For women over 60, it means building strength by starting with light weights and increasing as you get stronger. You can also improve endurance by walking longer or swimming harder. Flexibility increases, too, by stretching a bit more each time. It is important to listen to your body and not hurt yourself in the pursuit of pushing yourself to do more. Everyone improves at different speeds, so adjust exercises based on your fitness level and health. In addition, always focus on doing exercises safely to prevent injuries (Fischer, 2022).

Adaptation

Adaptation is your body adjusting to exercise. For women over 60, this means stronger muscles for better movement and balance. It also improves your heart and lung health, which is important for endurance. Plus, it helps keep your bones strong, reducing the risk of fractures. Give yourself time to rest between exercises. Rest days are crucial for your body to adapt to exercise. Besides, focus on exercises that help in daily activities like squats for sitting and standing up.

Monitoring Progress and Safety Measures

Track your progress by documenting your workouts in a journal or utilizing a fitness app. This practice not only maintains your motivation but also serves as a valuable reference tool. If you encounter difficulty with an exercise during the initial week of your fitness journey, make a note of it and attempt it again after a two-month interval.

Regularly review your fitness objectives and adapt your workout regimen every four to six weeks. Pay close attention to your body's signals and adjust exercise intensity accordingly. Note that fluctuations in your performance over time are normal; for instance, periods of illness may temporarily weaken your physical abilities. In such instances, it is advisable to regress to a comfortable level and gradually progress from there. Remember, achieving optimal fitness is a journey, not a sprint.

Emphasize proper exercise form to minimize the risk of injuries and optimize results. Gradual progression is key, so allocate ample time for rest and recovery between workout sessions.

Seeking Professional Guidance

Consistency in your workout routine is vital for progress. Choose enjoyable exercises to stay motivated, and remember to complement your training with a balanced diet and proper hydration. Following these guidelines, you can create a personalized strength training plan that meets your needs and boosts your overall well-being.

Understanding how aging affects the body and the role of strength training in counteracting these effects highlights the importance of assessing individual requirements before adding these exercises to your fitness regimen. Therefore, consulting a health care professional for any health or safety issues is necessary before developing a strength training plan. Once you have medical clearance and approval to start strength training, you can establish a tailored workout program. It's recommended to seek assistance from a certified personal trainer, especially if you're new to strength training, as they can provide advice on the correct form and design a customized workout routine.

Designing a workout plan that considers your fitness goals, abilities, and limitations is crucial for an effective routine. Specific steps need to be followed to craft a strength training plan aligned with your desired outcomes.

Strategies for Managing Soreness and Preventing Injury

Muscle soreness and injury prevention are major aspects of a fitness regimen. Sore muscles can hinder your ability to exercise and enjoy activities, while injuries can halt your progress and force you to take a break from training.

There are two types of muscle soreness to consider. Acute muscle soreness occurs during or immediately after exercise, often due to factors like the buildup of lactic acid. Fortunately, this soreness typically subsides within a few hours post-workout. Delayed onset muscle soreness (DOMS), on the other hand, arises 12–24 hours after physical activity and can last for 2–3 days. This type of soreness is caused by micro-tears in the muscles resulting from intense or novel activities, leading to stiffness and reduced mobility.

Several factors contribute to muscle soreness, and understanding these factors is essential for injury prevention. Eccentric contractions, where muscles lengthen while under tension, such as in downhill running or weight lifting, increase the likelihood of soreness by causing micro-tears. Intense workouts, sudden increases in exercise intensity, or engaging in unfamiliar activities can also result in prolonged soreness. Additionally, starting a new exercise routine or returning to workouts after a break can lead to sore muscles, as the body adjusts to new movement patterns (*Improving Health*, n.d.).

Various strategies can help alleviate muscle soreness. Prioritize a comprehensive warm-up involving light cardio and dynamic stretching before engaging in physical activity, and incorporate gentle exercises and static stretching into your post-workout routine to aid in recovery. It is advisable to gradually increase workout intensity to allow muscles to adapt properly. On rest days, engage in low-intensity activities like walking and consider massage therapy and hot–cold treatments for accelerated muscle recovery. In addition, consume protein-rich foods post-exercise to support muscle growth and repair, replenish energy stores with carbohydrate-rich foods, stay hydrated, ensure adequate sleep for recovery and overall health, and include rest days in your routine to prevent overexertion and reduce the risk of soreness and injuries (*Improving Health*, n.d.).

Preventing injury is exceptionally important as it can have serious and long-term repercussions. Thus, learn how to do exercises correctly to avoid getting hurt. Work on your core muscles and do functional exercises to improve your strength and balance, lowering your risk of injury. Additionally, stretch regularly and do mobility exercises to keep your joints and muscles moving well, reducing the chances of getting hurt.

SUMMARY

By slowly challenging their muscles and letting their bodies adapt, women over 60 can start a fitness journey that boosts strength, endurance, and overall health. Remember, stay consistent, be patient, and aim for gradual progress to achieve your fitness goals, no matter your age. Set realistic fitness goals based on what you like and need for your health, and keep track of your progress to see improvements over time. Furthermore, get advice from fitness experts or health care providers to create a personalized plan that considers any health issues.

7. WARM-UP MOVEMENTS

Prior to beginning strength training, it is essential to warm up, especially for women over 60, to ready the muscles, enhance flexibility, and lower the chances of injury. Here are some gentle yet effective warm-up routines:

Increase the heart rate and warm up lower-body muscles. Stand tall with feet hip-width apart. Commence marching in place, lifting knees comfortably high and swinging arms naturally. It is important to keep your breathing normal while completing this exercise.

Continue for two to three minutes.

Loosen shoulder joints and warm up upper-body muscles. Stand with feet shoulder-width apart, extend arms to the sides at shoulder height, and make small circles, gradually enlarging them. It is important to note that you must never push to a point of severe discomfort while warming up.

Continue for 30 seconds, then reverse for another 30 seconds.

Enhance hip mobility and warm up hip flexors and hamstrings. Stand next to a support wall or chair. Swing one leg forward and backward in a controlled manner. If you swing your leg around carelessly, you run the risk of pulling a muscle.

Perform 10–15 swings, then switch legs.

Loosen the spine and warm up core muscles. Stand with feet shoulder-width apart, hands on hips or extended out. Slowly twist your torso right and left while keeping your hips facing forward. Move as far as physically comfortable from side to side; this is a slow and controlled movement to avoid injury.

Perform 10–15 twists on each side.

Increase ankle joint mobility and warm up lower legs. Stand on one leg or sit for balance. Lift one foot and make ankle circles. You can use a wall to balance yourself; it is important not to lose balance and stumble, as this could lead to injury.

Perform 10–15 circles in each direction. Repeat on the other ankle.

Improve spine flexibility and warm up back muscles. You will need to use a yoga mat or a clean, dry surface for this warm-up exercise. Get on your hands and knees in the tabletop position. Inhale, arch back, and lift head and tailbone—cow pose. Exhale, round back, and tuck chin and tailbone—cat pose). It is once again important to not push yourself further than comfortable.

Repeat for 8–10 breaths, transitioning smoothly between poses.

Warm up shoulder muscles and boost blood flow to the upper body. Stand with feet shoulder-width apart, arms at sides. Lift shoulders toward ears, roll back and down. This is a movement that should be completed slowly and without straining yourself severely.

Perform 10–15 shrugs.

Utilize these guidelines for a safe and efficient warm-up.

- Allocate 5–10 minutes for proper preparation of muscles and joints.
- Maintain a consistent breathing pattern throughout the exercises.
- Start gently and escalate the intensity gradually.
- Be attentive and discontinue any exercise that induces pain or discomfort; opt for an alternative.

By incorporating these warm-up routines into your regime, you can guarantee a safe and productive strength training session, mitigating the risk of injuries and boosting performance levels.

8. Essential Strength Training Exercises

When planning to create your own strength training routine, it is important to add a variety of exercises. Adding a combination of upper-body, lower-body, and core exercises in a routine is imperative, as you must work out all of your muscles.

Here are a few practical tips before trying the exercises:

- Remove rings—holding a weight will hurt your fingers—and any other jewelry that will get in your way while exercising.
- Ensure you have all the necessary equipment.
- Remember that you can use alternative equipment; for example, if you do not have dumbbells, you can use a filled water bottle.
- Wear items like exercise gloves and sneakers for extra grip.
- Wear items like knee pads for extra padding.
- Do not make any fast movements; move slowly into each exercise, and remember to breathe properly.

- Have a bottle of water as well as a chair within reachable distance.
- Above all else, listen to your body if you feel any sharp pain or discomfort. Stop the movement immediately, and take a moment to rest and reassess if you have an injury.

It is important to understand what muscles will be activated with each different exercise.

UPPER-BODY EXERCISES

Bicep Curls

- Difficulty: *
- Why: The bicep, a vital muscle for lifting, carrying, holding, and reaching, is strengthened effectively through bicep curls.
- Instructions: Position yourself with feet shoulder-width apart. Grasp a dumbbell in each hand, ensuring your arms are fully extended. Raise the weights toward your shoulders while keeping your elbows close to your sides. Lower the dumbbells back down methodically, avoiding any swinging motion, and concentrate on moving the weights with precise control.
- Adaptions: Sit on a backless chair if prolonged standing is challenging. Perform the exercise without dumbbells or opt for a lighter dumbbell for better practice.

Shoulder Presses

- Difficulty: *
- Why: Shoulder presses target the deltoid and triceps muscles, improving shoulder mobility and strength for lifting, carrying, and reaching tasks.
- Instructions: Sit or stand with your feet shoulder-width apart. Hold a dumbbell in each hand at shoulder level with palms facing forward. Push the weights upward and then lower them down. Remember to tighten your core to maintain proper posture and perform the full motion to engage muscles effectively.
- Adaptions: Sit on a chair without armrests if prolonged standing is challenging. Practice the exercise without dumbbells or with a lighter dumbbell.

Chest Press

- Difficulty: **
- Why: It enhances your capacity to exert force, whether lifting yourself from the ground or moving a shopping cart. Target your chest, triceps, and shoulders with the chest press exercise.
- Instructions: Begin by lying on a bench with your feet flat on the floor. Start without weights, focusing on proper form. If you are ready to add dumbbells, increase the weight slowly by gripping a dumbbell in each hand at chest level to ensure you do not overexert yourself. Press the dumbbells upward until your arms are fully extended, then lower them back down. Maintain a neutral wrist position and keep your shoulder blades against the bench throughout the movement.

- Adaptions: Adjust your bench or couch to a 45° incline angle. Perform the exercise without any dumbbells initially, or start with a lighter dumbbell for practice.

Bent-Over Rows

- Difficulty: **
- Why: Strengthen your back muscles effectively while enhancing trunk and hip stability. Engage your back muscles with bent-over rows.
- Instructions: Stand with feet shoulder-width apart, knees slightly bent. Bend at the hips, maintain a straight back, and grasp a dumbbell in each hand. Draw the weights toward your torso, your elbows close to your body. Keep your back straight, avoid hunching, and contract your shoulder blades together at the movement's peak.
- Adaptions: Perform a row using one arm at a time, resting your opposite hand on a bench for stability. You can also position yourself face-down on an adjustable bench at a slight incline, allowing the dumbbells to hang directly down with extended arms, your palms turned toward each other. Pull upward in a slow, strong movement.

Tricep Dips

- Difficulty: *
- Why: Enhances flexibility and boosts the capacity to lift yourself up, for instance, from a sofa or seat. Strengthen your triceps, shoulders, and chest effectively with tricep dips.
- Instructions: Position your hands on a bench or parallel bars while keeping your legs extended. Lower your body by bending your elbows and then push back up. Keep your

back straight and your arms to your sides; avoid excessive dipping to prevent strain on your shoulders.

- Adaptions: Perform the exercise to a point where you can feel your triceps engaging. As you develop strength, you'll find yourself able to increase your movement's depth. Adjust the difficulty level by positioning your feet closer to your body with bent legs for an easier variation or placing your feet farther away for a more challenging version.

Lat Pull-Downs

- Difficulty: *
- Why: The lat pull-down exercise primarily targets the latissimus dorsi muscles, known as the lats, extending from the mid to the side of the back. It also engages the shoulder, arm, and core muscles. Furthermore, as the lifter pulls the bar down toward the chest, the biceps and forearms become also actively involved. Thus, it is an exercise that focuses on the entire upper body.
- Instructions: Engage your back muscles, biceps, and shoulders by sitting at a lat pull-down machine and gripping the bar widely. If a lat pull-down machine is unavailable, utilize dumbbells or filled water bottles to modify the exercise. Pull the bar down toward your chest, focusing on squeezing your shoulder blades together, and then return it to the starting position. Emphasize using your back muscles and avoid relying on momentum to bring the bar down.
- Adaptions:

  - Supinated grip: Palms facing away from you.
  - Pronated grip: Palms facing toward you.
  - Narrow grip: Grasping the bar closer to the center.

    o Wide grip: Grasping the bar at the ends.

Push-Ups

- Difficulty: **
- Why: Boost muscle growth and enhance upper-body strength by specifically targeting the pectoralis major in the chest, the triceps in the arms, and the scapular stabilizing muscles in the shoulders.
- Instructions: Performing push-ups activates multiple muscle groups simultaneously, including the chest, triceps, shoulders, and core. Commence in a plank position with hands positioned slightly wider than shoulder-width. Lower your body until your chest is near the ground, then push up. Ensure your body maintains alignment, and actively engage your core muscles throughout the entire movement.
- Adaptions: Get into a hands-and-knees position, with your gaze toward the floor. Position your hands a bit wider than your shoulders and space your knees comfortably apart.

Lateral Raises

- Difficulty: *
- Why: Target your shoulder muscles with lateral raises, which not only enhance your physical appearance but also boost shoulder mobility, improve range of motion, and enhance stability.
- Instructions: Position yourself with feet shoulder-width apart. Lift the weights sideways until your arms are level with the ground. Slowly return the weights to the starting position, maintaining a slight elbow bend throughout the exercise to avoid momentum.

- Adaptations: Engage your elbows in a slight bend before starting the exercise. This modified lateral raise with bent arms reduces the distance of the weight from your body as you move.

Pull-Ups

- Difficulty: ***
- Why: Strengthen your arm, shoulder, and back muscles with this effective exercise that enhances overall body strength and fitness.
- Instructions: Engage in pull-ups to effectively target your back, biceps, and shoulders. Hang from the bar using an overhand grip, pulling your body upward until your chin surpasses the bar. Lower your body down with controlled movements, and focus on core engagement to prevent any swinging.
- Adaptations:

  ○ Perform an assisted pull-up by securing a resistance band around the pull-up bar. Position one or both feet or knees on the band based on its length and tightness. Execute a traditional pull-up following proper form, letting the band assist you as you raise your head above the bar. Concentrate on mastering the correct movement pattern.
  ○ For a chin-up, stand on a bench or jump box beneath the pull-up bar. Grip the bar with both hands in a palm-up position. Similar to a pull-up form, elevate your chest toward the bar, briefly pausing at the top before slowly lowering back to the initial position. Although resembling pull-ups, chin-ups impact the body differently due to variations in grip and movement.

○ In a seated pull-up, begin seated with legs extended and a pull-up bar conveniently overhead. Place your heels on a small box or bench. Maintain traditional pull-up form, bending elbows to lift your body until your chin surpasses the bar. Apply additional force through your feet if required, gradually lowering back to the seated position.

Plank Rows–Renegade Rows

- Difficulty: ****
- Why: Enhances strength in the mid- and upper-back area while improving stability throughout the spine and shoulders. Engage various muscle groups, including the back, shoulders, biceps, and core, by performing plank rows.
- Instructions: Initiate the exercise in a plank stance, grasping a dumbbell in each hand. Elevate one weight toward your side while preserving stability in your body, then return it downward and repeat the motion using the alternate arm. Ensure your hips remain level to prevent any rotation and uphold a robust plank form throughout the activity.
- Adaption: Begin in an adapted push-up position with knees and hands instead of a traditional plank pose.

LOWER-BODY EXERCISES

Squats

- Difficulty: ***
- Why: Squats engage the quadriceps, hamstrings, glutes, and calves, enhancing core strength and leg muscle development, thus boosting bone health, flexibility, and overall athletic performance.
- Instructions: To perform a squat, position your feet shoulder-width apart. Bend your knees and hips, lowering your body until your thighs are parallel to the ground. Maintain a straight back throughout the movement. Drive through your heels to return to the standing position. Ensure your knees align with your toes and avoid inward movement.
- Adaptations:

  - Wall squat: The wall squat is a great exercise for working out your legs. To do a wall squat, you simply stand with your back against the wall and lower yourself into a sitting position. Keep your feet shoulder-width apart and your back straight against the wall. Hold the position for a few seconds before pushing yourself back up to standing. This exercise helps strengthen your quadriceps, hamstrings, and glutes. It's a good way to build endurance and improve your overall leg strength.
  - Sit-to-stand squat: The sit-to-stand squat is another effective exercise that targets multiple muscle groups. Start by sitting in a chair with your feet flat on the floor. Stand up from the chair using only your leg muscles, then slowly lower yourself back down. This exercise is

great for improving your lower-body strength, especially in your thighs and glutes. It also helps with balance and coordination. Try doing several sets of sit-to-stand squats to feel the burn in your legs.

- o Stand-to-sit squat: The stand-to-sit squat is similar to the sit-to-stand squat but in reverse. Begin by standing in front of a chair with your feet hip-width apart. Slowly lower yourself into a seated position on the chair, then stand back up using your leg muscles. This exercise is beneficial for strengthening your leg muscles and improving your ability to sit and stand with ease. It also works your core muscles as you stabilize your body during the movements. Practice stand-to-sit squats regularly to enhance your lower-body strength.

Incorporating these three types of squats into your workout routine can help you achieve stronger and more toned legs. Remember to maintain proper form while performing these exercises to prevent injury and maximize their benefits. Start with a few repetitions and gradually increase the intensity as your strength improves. Stay consistent with your workouts to see progress over time.

Lunges

- Difficulty: ***
- Why: Engaging in lunges as part of one's workout regimen is certain to enhance both posture and flexibility. Lunges focus on strengthening the quadriceps, hamstrings, and glutes.
- Instructions: To execute a lunge, position your feet hip-width apart. Take a step forward with one leg, bending both knees to 90° angles. Return to the initial stance and

switch legs. Maintain an upright posture and ensure the front knee does not extend beyond the toes.
- Adaptions:

  ○ Stabilized lunge: In this lunge variation, you utilize a fixed object like a wall or chair to enhance your stability. This allows you to concentrate on your posture without the concern of leaning to either side. Place your palm on the object to steady yourself as you lower and raise yourself up.
  ○ Partial lunge: This version entails a reduced range of motion as you descend only half the distance compared to a regular lunge, halting well before your leading knee reaches a 90° angle. This can aid in maintaining proper form while minimizing the pressure on the knee joints.

Dead Lifts

- Difficulty: **
- Why: Strengthening your back and core muscles enhances your speed directly. Dead lifts target your hamstrings, glutes, and lower back.
- Instructions: Initiate the deadlift by positioning your feet hip-width apart and the barbell in front of you. Hinge at your hips and knees to grip the barbell with an overhand hold. Elevate the barbell by extending your hips and knees while maintaining a flat back. Lower the bar in proximity to your body, ensuring your back remains unrounded.
- Adaptations: Resistance bands and chains provide adjustable levels of resistance during the dead lift movement, offering varying challenges to weight lifters.

Glute Bridges

- Difficulty: ***
- Why: Glute bridges target and strengthen the gluteal muscles, hamstrings, and lower back. These exercises improve hip stability, enhance athletic performance, and alleviate lower-back discomfort.
- Instruction: Lie on your back with your knees bent and feet flat on the floor. Raise your hips until your body forms a straight line, and tighten your glute muscles at the top. Ensure not to arch your lower back, and concentrate on engaging your glutes.
- Adaptations: Place a dumbbell or weighted bag on your hips to start. Secure the weight as you raise and lower your hips to prevent it from slipping or rolling off. Engage in single-leg bridges. To enhance stability, aim to not only target your glutes but also challenge your core muscles further.

Step-Ups

- Difficulty: **
- Why: Step-ups target and strengthen your quadriceps, hamstrings, glutes, and legs.
- Instructions: Stand facing a bench or step. Step up with one leg, bringing the other up to stand on the bench. Step back down, alternating legs, and maintain control of your movements. Ensure your entire foot is on the bench for stability.
- Adaptations: Elevate the workout by grasping dumbbells or opting for a taller step.

Bulgarian Split Squats

- Difficulty: ***
- Why: Bulgarian split squats target the quadriceps, hamstrings, and glutes effectively.
- Instructions: Place one foot on the bench behind you. Lower your body until your front thigh is parallel to the ground, then push back up, ensuring your upper body remains upright. Be mindful not to let your front knee extend beyond your toes.
- Adaptions: Position yourself with one foot forward about 2 ft ahead, adjusting the distance according to your limb proportions if needed. Ensure the ball of your rear foot remains firmly on the ground. Use the hand on the opposite side of your active leg to grip a stable surface like a chair's back, a squat rack's post, or secure gymnastics rings. Lower yourself slowly until your back knee lightly touches the ground or hovers approximately 1 in. above it. If your knee touches down, prevent it from crashing too forcefully. To rise back up, press through your front foot while avoiding raising onto your toes or over-relying on your back foot.

Calf Raises

- Difficulty: *
- Why: Calf raises target your calf muscles, which are important for walking, bending, etc.
- Instructions: Position your feet hip-width apart and elevate your heels, balancing on the balls of your feet. Gradually lower your heels to the starting position, ensuring a full range of motion. If necessary, you may utilize a support for stability.

- Adaptations: Perform single-leg calf raises or utilize a step to enhance the range of motion.

Leg Press

- Difficulty: **
- Why: The leg press exercises your quadriceps, hamstrings, and glutes.
- Instructions: Position yourself on the leg press machine, ensuring your feet are shoulder-width apart on the platform. Push the platform forward by straightening your knees and hips, then return gradually to the initial position. Maintain a flat back against the seat and refrain from fully straightening your knees during the exercise.
- Adaptations: Adjust your foot positioning on the platform to target specific muscle groups or decrease resistance by removing the weights.

Romanian Dead Lifts

- Difficulty: ***
- Why: Romanian dead lifts target your hamstrings, glutes, and lower back.
- Instructions: Position your feet hip-width apart and grasp a barbell or dumbbell. Hinge at your hips while ensuring your back remains in a straight line, then return to the initial position by thrusting your hips forward. Keep the weights near your body and sustain a neutral spine throughout the exercise.
- Adaptations: Utilize resistance bands or chains for varied resistance levels throughout the entire range of motion.

Hip Thrusts

- Difficulty: ***
- Why: Hip thrusts work your glutes, hamstrings, and lower back.
- Instructions: Sit on the ground, back against a bench, feet flat. Place a barbell over your hips and raise them until your body is straight, maintaining glute contractions and a tucked chin throughout.
- Adaptations: Secure a resistance band around your thighs to enhance glute activation, or engage in single-leg hip thrusts for a more challenging workout.

Core Exercises

Planks

- Difficulty: **
- Why: Planks are a great exercise for your core, shoulders, and back.
- Instructions: Perform a plank by assuming a push-up stance while supporting your body weight on your forearms. Ensure your body forms a straight line from head to heels. Activate your core muscles to uphold proper alignment and prevent your hips from either dropping or lifting. Maintain a consistent breathing pattern throughout the exercise duration.
- Adaptations: Enhance the challenge by raising one leg or one arm or executing side planks to specifically target your oblique muscles.

Abdominal Crunches

- Difficulty: *
- Why: Abdominal crunches mainly target your upper abdominals. Strengthening your core is important for stability.
- Instructions: Position your body on your back, bending the knees and placing your hands behind your head. Elevate your shoulders from the ground while ensuring your lower back remains firm against the floor. Avoid straining your neck and concentrate on deliberate movements to effectively activate your abdominal muscles.
- Adaptations: Strengthen your obliques by placing a weight on your chest or doing bicycle crunches.

Bicycle Crunches

- Difficulty: **
- Why: Bicycle crunches work your abdominal muscles and obliques.
- Instructions: Lie on your back with knees bent and hands behind your head. Elevate your shoulders and rotate your torso to draw one knee toward your chest as you stretch the opposing leg. Ensure deliberate, unhurried movements, concentrating on the rotational aspect of your midsection.

Leg Raises

- Difficulty: **
- Why: Leg raises target your lower abdominals and hip flexors.

- Instructions: Lie on your back with legs extended upward, raise them to a vertical position, and lower them back down slowly without touching the ground, ensuring controlled movements while keeping your lower back firmly against the floor.
- Adaptations: Perform the exercise with legs bent at the knee to alleviate the pressure.

Russian Twists

- Difficulty: **
- Why: Russian twists engage your obliques and abdominals.
- Instructions: Sit on the ground with knees bent and feet flat and lifted off the ground. Hold a weight or medicine ball and twist your torso from side to side. Remember to keep your core engaged and your back straight, avoiding excessive use of your arms.
- Adaptations: Increase the difficulty by using a heavier weight or extending your legs straight out.

Mountain Climbers

- Difficulty: **
- Why: Mountain climbers work your abdominals, hip flexors, and shoulders.
- Instructions: Begin in a plank position and alternate by bringing each knee toward your chest rapidly. Engage your core throughout to prevent hips from dropping, and maintain a consistent speed during the exercise.
- Adaptations: Bring your legs up in a slow, controlled movement and lower repetitions to lighten the workout.

Dead Bug

- Difficulty: **
- Why: The dead bug exercise targets your abdominals and hip flexors.
- Instructions: While lying on your back, extend your arms toward the ceiling and bend your knees at a 90° angle. Slowly lower one arm and the opposite leg toward the ground, then return to the starting position. Focus on controlled movements and keeping your lower back flat on the floor.

Side Planks

- Difficulty: **
- Why: Side planks are effective for working your obliques, shoulders, and core.
- Instructions: When performing side planks, position yourself on one side with your elbow aligned under your shoulder. Elevate your hips to create a straight line, maintaining a rigid body position without allowing your hips to drop.
- Adaptations: Hold the position for a few moments instead of moving up and down.

Hanging Leg Raises

- Difficulty: ***
- Why: Hanging leg raises focus on your lower abdominals and hip flexors.
- Instructions: Grip the pull-up bar with arms fully extended and lift your legs toward your chest in a

controlled motion, ensuring they remain steady without swinging. Engage your core muscles to effortlessly raise your legs upward.

- Adaptations: Perform the exercise with legs bent at the knee to alleviate the pressure.

Reverse Crunches

- Difficulty: **
- Why: Reverse crunches target the lower abdominals.
- Instructions: Lie flat on your back, bend your knees, and lift your feet off the ground. Support your hips by placing your hands underneath, then raise them off the ground. Focus on deliberate movements and continuously engage your lower abdominal muscles throughout the exercise.
- Adaptations: Raise your legs only as far as physically comfortable; you do not have to lift your legs all the way up.

MODIFICATIONS AND VARIATIONS FOR DIFFERENT FITNESS LEVELS AND ABILITIES

Strength training or any exercise should be adaptable to suit different fitness levels and abilities so that everyone can participate safely and effectively. The adjustments are vital to ensure individuals with varying strengths and flexibility can engage in physical activities regardless of their starting point. Let's delve into how modifications and variations cater to different needs.

Modifications

- Reduced intensity: Beginners should initiate their fitness journey with lighter weights, resistance bands, or body weight exercises to gradually build strength and enhance technique. Conversely, seasoned practitioners have the option to elevate resistance levels or introduce more demanding movements to challenge their muscles effectively.

- Simplified movements: Newcomers should prioritize mastering fundamental exercise variations with basic movements to focus on perfecting form and technique. Conversely, individuals at an advanced level can delve into more complex movements or progressive variations to heighten intensity and refine skills.

- Assisted movements: New individuals may benefit from utilizing tools such as stability balls or chairs and seeking guidance from trainers to enhance their balance and stability during exercises. More experienced individuals may prefer focusing on exercises that do not rely on external support, aiming to enhance core stability and refine muscle control.

- Range of motion adjustments: For beginners, it's advisable to adjust the range of motion to a comfortable level to avoid strain and injury. On the other hand, advanced individuals may find increasing the range of motion beneficial for fully engaging muscles and improving flexibility.

Variations

- Equipment options: Beginners should start with basic gym equipment or minimal gear like resistance bands. In contrast, advanced individuals can opt for specialized equipment such as barbells, kettlebells, or gym machines to introduce additional resistance and challenge purposes.

- Body positioning: For beginners, exercises in stable positions like seated or lying down provide safety and comfort. Advanced practitioners can advance their balance and coordination by trying exercises in dynamic positions, such as standing or on unstable surfaces.
- Tempo and speed: Beginners should prioritize deliberate and precise movements to cultivate muscle coordination and minimize the likelihood of injury. Those at an advanced level can integrate rapid tempos or plyometric workouts to amplify the strength and endurance of the muscles.
- Integration of variations: Beginners should start with basic exercises they can handle. Over time, they can gradually introduce more challenging options as their fitness levels increase. Those more experienced rotate through a variety of advanced variations to keep progress steady and consistently push their physical limits.

Importance of Modifications and Variations

- Safety: Minimizing the chances of workout-related injuries; particularly beneficial for novices or those with physical constraints.
- Progression: Enabling individuals to commence training at their present fitness level and incrementally intensify their regimen as they enhance their strength and abilities.
- Inclusivity: Ensuring fitness is within reach for individuals of varying abilities, ages, or health conditions, encouraging participation in fitness initiatives.
- Personalization: Customizing workout routines to cater to specific requirements and maximizing outcomes and enjoyment by proposing alternatives aligned with personal fitness aspirations and capabilities.

By incorporating adjustments and variations into strength training or any workout program, individuals can significantly boost their physical capabilities and fitness levels, and accomplish their health goals in a safe and sustainable manner.

9. Advanced Training Techniques

Incorporating Resistance Bands, Stability Balls, and Other Equipment

Using tools like resistance bands, stability balls, and other equipment can greatly boost the effectiveness and enjoyment of strength training. These versatile instruments provide various advantages, making workouts more accessible, adaptable, and engaging.

Resistance Bands

Resistance bands provide adjustable resistance levels for various workouts that target specific muscle groups. Unlike traditional weights, the consistent resistance offered by bands boosts muscle activation and endurance. Their customizable design accommodates individuals of different strength levels by allowing adjustments to the band or grip position, making them suitable for both novices and seasoned fitness enthusiasts.

Resistance bands offer unparalleled portability, making them a perfect choice for home, travel, or outdoor workouts. With their compact and lightweight design, women can effortlessly maintain their strength training routine without the need for a full gym setup. This convenience fosters dedication and consistency in adhering to their fitness regimen.

Furthermore, the controlled resistance offered by resistance bands is gentle on the joints in comparison to traditional weights. This aspect specifically benefits older individuals with joint issues or those recovering from injuries. The bands' elasticity facilitates smooth, deliberate movements, thereby minimizing the chance of injury while effectively activating the muscles (*Resistance Bands*, n.d.).

Stability Balls

Stability balls are effective tools for enhancing core strength and stability. Exercising on an unstable surface like a stability ball activates various stabilizing muscles to maintain balance. This dynamic engagement strengthens the core muscles and improves overall stability and coordination, which is essential for preventing falls and maintaining functional fitness in daily life.

Using a stability ball can improve flexibility and increase the range of motion. The ball allows for dynamic stretching and movements that cannot be achieved on flat surfaces, which can greatly help older individuals maintain joint health and mobility, thus enhancing their ability to perform daily activities with ease.

Moreover, stability balls provide diverse exercise options, acting as back support for core workouts, adding balance to strength training, and aiding in stretching routines. Their versatility makes them a vital part of any workout routine, offering a wide range of choices to keep the workout engaging and challenging (Thompson, 2023).

Other Equipment

Light Dumbbells and Ankle Weights

Small weights and ankle bands serve as valuable tools for elevating resistance in a variety of workout routines, aiding in the development of muscle strength and endurance. These pieces of equipment are especially beneficial for strengthening specific muscles and crucial for preserving muscle mass and bone density. Their customizable design enables gradual advancement, suiting diverse strength levels and fitness objectives (Castro-Sloboda, n.d.).

Foam Rollers

Foam rollers are vital for aiding in muscle recovery and enhancing flexibility. They serve the purpose of self-myofascial release, easing muscle tightness, boosting blood circulation, and promoting muscle recovery. Incorporating foam rollers into a regular fitness regimen can help prevent injuries and advance overall flexibility, making them an essential component of a holistic fitness routine (Elliott, n.d.).

Balance Boards

Elderly individuals can enhance their balance and coordination using balance boards that are necessary for preventing falls and maintaining independence. Training on these boards activates core muscles and stabilizers, improving overall stability and body awareness and leading to enhanced performance in exercises and daily tasks (*Balance Boards*, 2021).

Summary

Incorporating resistance bands, stability balls, and other equipment into strength training for women over 60 offers various benefits. These tools provide adaptability and joint-friendly resistance, making strength training more accessible and effective. In addition, they boost core strength, balance, flexibility, and overall muscle conditioning, enhancing health and functional fitness. By including these tools in their workouts, women can have a diverse and engaging fitness routine that supports their well-being in later years.

EXPLORING DIFFERENT TRAINING MODALITIES

As women age, it's essential to combine diverse training methods to uphold dynamic, efficient workouts that align precisely with their fitness goals. Experimenting with various training techniques, such as circuit training and interval training, can yield numerous benefits and enhance the overall workout experience.

Circuit Training

Circuit training consists of "a series of exercises performed consecutively with minimal rest between each." This workout method combines strength and cardiovascular exercises, providing a thorough and time-efficient fitness routine.

Circuit training offers numerous benefits, especially for those with limited time. By incorporating both strength and cardio elements, it delivers a comprehensive workout in a short duration. The diverse range of movements not only maintains engagement but also reduces monotony, encouraging consistent dedication to the fitness regimen. Moreover, including activities that mimic daily tasks can improve functional fitness and simplify everyday activities. In addition, integrating strength and cardio exercises raises the heart rate and boosts calorie burn, aiding in weight management and overall health. Additionally, circuit training is highly adaptable to different fitness levels and can utilize various equipment such as resistance bands, stability balls, and light dumbbells (Robinson, 2014).

Interval Training

Interval training involves alternating between high-intensity exercise and periods of lower intensity or rest. This technique benefits cardiovascular and strength training programs. Furthermore, interval training is essential for heart health and highly effective in improving cardiovascular fitness compared to steady-state cardio.

By including high-intensity intervals, it boosts metabolism, leading to increased calorie expenditure during and after workouts. The mix of high and low intensity enables individuals to handle a more significant workout load, enhancing endurance and muscle strength simultaneously. Similar to circuit training in terms of time efficiency, interval training offers a powerful workout in a shorter duration. The varying intensity levels create an engaging workout experience, boosting motivation and consistency significantly (Walker, 2008).

Combining Training Modalities

Utilizing a diverse range of training methods offers a comprehensive approach to fitness. For instance, integrating circuit training and interval training into a weekly regimen can optimize the advantages of each method while maintaining variety and excitement in workouts.

Women aged 60 and above can personalize their workout routines based on their fitness levels, objectives, and preferences. For example, an individual might opt for circuit training due to its all-encompassing nature and interval training for its cardiovascular advantages. Adapting the exercises to suit specific requirements guarantees a well-rounded and efficient fitness program.

In summary, a well-rounded workout regimen involves a mix of strength training, cardiovascular exercises, and flexibility training. This diverse method enhances muscle strength, heart health, flexibility, and overall fitness levels.

Safety and Considerations

Women over 60 are advised to consult with fitness professionals when exploring new training methods. Seeking guidance from your health care provider or certified trainers can help create personalized workout plans, ensuring correct form and technique and making necessary adjustments to accommodate physical limitations or health issues.

Listen to your body during your workout routine, and avoid pushing yourself too hard. Pay close attention to how your body reacts to various exercises and levels of intensity, and make adjustments as needed. Remember, taking time to rest and recover is just as important as exercising to prevent injuries and maintain long-term fitness.

Begin with easier exercises and progressively elevate the challenge and intricacy. This method enables the body to adjust and minimizes the risk of injury. Note that it is crucial to establish a firm groundwork before advancing to more demanding workout routines.

Exploring various training methods like circuit training and interval training can greatly enhance the strength training experience for women aged 60 and above. These methods bring multiple advantages, including improved heart health, increased strength and endurance, time efficiency, and higher engagement levels. By integrating a range of training techniques, women can establish a well-rounded, enjoyable, and efficient fitness routine that promotes their health and overall well-being. With expert supervision and a strong emphasis on safety, these training methods can assist women over 60 in reaching their fitness objectives and sustaining an active, healthy lifestyle.

CROSS-TRAINING AND ITS BENEFITS FOR OVERALL FITNESS AND INJURY PREVENTION

For women aged 60 and above, integrating cross-training into their fitness regimen can offer a comprehensive approach to exercise, improving overall physical fitness and lowering the risk of injuries. Discover the numerous benefits cross-training offers and learn how to infuse it seamlessly into your workout schedule. Cross-training entails diversifying your exercise routine by engaging in a variety of activities, ensuring the engagement of different muscle groups and reaping the benefits of a wide spectrum of physical exercises. Women in the 60 and above age bracket can embrace cross-training by fusing strength training, cardiovascular workouts, flexibility exercises, and balance enhancement exercises.

Benefits of Cross-Training

Engage in diverse exercises to strengthen all major muscle groups, achieving a well-rounded and sculpted physique. Incorporating cardio activities like walking, swimming, or cycling enhances heart health and endurance, complementing the muscle gains from strength training. Cross-training facilitates recovery of different muscle groups while you target others, decreasing the risk of overuse injuries. Moreover, diversifying your workouts can prevent strain on joints, which is vital for sustaining joint health and warding off conditions such as arthritis. By altering your routine, you can maintain excitement in exercise and avoid monotony, making the experience enjoyable and motivating. In addition, embracing new activities adds a fresh challenge and keeps your mental acuity sharp. Introducing activities like yoga or Pilates enhances flexibility, which is essential for daily functions and preventing rigidity. On the other hand, engaging in exercises focusing on balance, such as tai chi, aids in preventing falls and enhancing stability. Pursuing activities like yoga and tai chi also confers mental well-being benefits, reducing stress and promoting relaxation. Additionally, joining group classes or fitness communities fosters social interaction and aid, which is vital for mental well-being (*Cross Training*, n.d.).

How to Incorporate Cross-Training

- Establish a well-balanced weekly routine: Engage in strength training two to three times per week, focusing on all major muscle groups. Allocate a day of rest between sessions for optimal muscle recovery.
- Cardiovascular workouts: Aim for a minimum of 150 minutes of moderate-intensity cardio each week, such as brisk walking, swimming, cycling, or dancing.
- Enhance flexibility and balance: Integrate flexibility and balance exercises into your routine two to three times weekly, with options like yoga, Pilates, and tai chi being highly beneficial.

Sample Weekly Plan

- Monday: Strength training (upper body)
- Tuesday: Cardio (brisk walking) + flexibility (yoga)
- Wednesday: Strength training (lower body)
- Thursday: Cardio (swimming) + balance (tai chi)
- Friday: Strength training (full body)
- Saturday: Cardio (cycling) + flexibility (stretching)
- Sunday: Rest or light activity (gentle stretching or a leisurely walk)

Listen to Your Body

Listen to your body's signals and adjust your routine accordingly. If you feel any pain or discomfort, make changes to the exercise or allow yourself a day of rest.

Ensure you give your body enough time to recover between rigorous workouts to avoid overtraining and potential injuries.

Seek Professional Guidance

Engage a certified personal trainer with expertise in training older adults to devise a tailored cross-training regimen aligned with your specific requirements and objectives. Participate in fitness classes supervised by proficient instructors to ensure correct and safe execution of exercises.

Cross-training, a flexible and efficient fitness strategy, yields manifold benefits for women aged 60 and above. By integrating various exercises into your regimen, you can enhance overall fitness levels, diminish injury risks, and derive greater enjoyment and motivation from your workout routine. Remember, the fundamental elements of successful cross-training comprise equilibrium, diversity, and attentiveness to your body's cues. Through a comprehensive fitness blueprint, you can attain your health and wellness aspirations, preserve self-reliance, and embrace an active and gratifying lifestyle.

10. Cooldown Movements

Spend at least 5–10 minutes cooling down to ensure your heart rate and breathing return to normal and your muscles relax. Focus on deep, controlled breathing to promote relaxation and reduce muscle tension. Perform stretches slowly and gently, avoiding any fast or sudden movements.

By incorporating these cooldown exercises into your routine, you can help ensure a safe and effective transition from exercise to rest, reducing the risk of injury and promoting overall flexibility and relaxation. Cooldown exercises help reduce sore muscles and quicken muscle repair.

- walking or marching in place

  - Walk or march in place at a gentle, consistent pace. Concentrate on deep, steady breathing. This will relax your leg muscles.
  - Continue for two to three minutes.

- seated forward bend

  - This extends the hamstrings, lower back, and calves. Sit on the floor with your legs stretched out in front of you. Slowly lean forward from the hips, reaching toward your toes. Do not push yourself to stretch further than is comfortable. This is a cooldown, not an exercise, so it is meant to calm down your muscles. Maintain the stretch for 20–30 seconds, then return to the starting position slowly.
  - Repeat two to three times.

- chest opener stretch:

  - It stretches the chest and shoulders. Stand with feet shoulder-width apart. If you are able to, clasp your hands behind your back and gently raise your arms, expanding your chest. If you are unable to do this, stretch your arms out toward your sides, stretching your arms as far back as comfortable. Hold for 20–30 seconds while breathing deeply.
  - Release and repeat two to three times.

- quadriceps stretch

  - Targets the front thigh muscles–quadriceps. Stand near a wall or chair for support. Bend one knee, bringing the heel toward the buttocks. Hold the ankle with your hand and gently pull toward the buttocks.
  - Maintain the stretch for 20–30 seconds. Repeat with the other leg.

- calf stretch

  - Stretches the calf muscles. Face a wall with hands at shoulder height on the wall. Step one foot back, keeping the heel down and the back leg straight. Slightly bend the front knee and lean forward until feeling the calf stretch in the back leg.
  - Hold for 20–30 seconds. Repeat on the other leg.

- seated spinal twist

  - Stretches back muscles and enhances spinal flexibility. Sit on the floor with your legs extended. Bend your right knee, placing the foot on the outside of your left thigh. Put your left hand on the right knee and the right hand behind for support. Gently twist your torso to the right, looking over your shoulder.
  - Hold the stretch for 20–30 seconds. Repeat on the other side.

- overhead arm stretch

  - Stretches upper back and shoulders. Stand or sit with feet shoulder-width apart. Raise one arm overhead and bend the elbow, reaching down your back. Use the other hand to press down gently on the bent elbow.
  - Hold for 20–30 seconds. Repeat on the other arm.

- cat-cow stretch

  - Increases flexibility and stretches the spine. Position hands and knees in a tabletop stance. Inhale, arch your back, and raise your head and tailbone toward the

ceiling—cow pose. Exhale, round your back, and tuck your chin and tailbone toward your chest—cat pose.
  ○ Repeat for 8–10 breaths, transitioning smoothly between poses.

Be aware of your body's signals during the cooldown. Stop any stretch causing pain and try a different movement. Incorporating these cooldown exercises fosters a safe and effective transition from exercise to rest, lowering injury risk and enhancing flexibility and relaxation overall.

11. Creating a Safe and Supportive Workout Environment

Embarking on a fresh workout regimen can feel overwhelming, particularly when delving into the realm of strength training. Enter this guide: Establishing a strong foundation and grasping key elements are crucial for a seamless commencement of this new journey. By this stage, you have assessed your fitness level, familiarized yourself with warm-up, cooldown, and essential exercises, comprehended the significance of strength training, and constructed a personalized workout plan.

Now, it is time to prime your workout environment since it is important to prep this environment for a variety of reasons.

Prepare your workout space by organizing your equipment for easy access and ensuring no obstacles could lead to injuries. Prioritize safety in your home workout area by using a nonslip mat and clearing the space for unrestricted movement. Regularly inspect your gear to maintain its quality. Select appropriate equipment tailored to your fitness level, such as light dumbbells, resistance bands, and stability balls for strength training, offering a safer alternative to heavy weights. Opt for adjustable weights to progressively increase the intensity of your workouts.

Before and following exercise, it is essential to warm up and cool down to maintain muscle wellness (*Warm Up, Cool Down*, 2014). To warm up, engage in light activities such as walking or cycling for a few minutes to boost blood circulation. Incorporating dynamic stretching, which involves stretching during movement, is beneficial for priming your body. Following your workout, gradually lower your heart rate through gentle cooldown exercises. Utilizing static stretching aids in muscle relaxation and elongation, decreasing soreness. Establish a routine of warming up and cooling down each time you work out. This practice assists in injury prevention and enhances overall performance.

A safe workout environment is not only about having the physical location prepped but also how well-informed you are before commencing the workout routine.

Being on your own side is vital. Just as important as working out is taking breaks. It's essential to give your muscles time to heal so you can continue on a slow and steady pace, without any setbacks. Make sure to include scheduled *rest days* in your routine. By allowing your muscles one or two days of rest each week, you are aiding in their repair and strengthening. On these rest days, engage in light activities such as walking or gentle yoga to promote blood flow and muscle recovery without overexerting yourself. Listen to your body during and after workouts; if you feel very fatigued or experience pain, consider slowing down or taking an extended break. Understanding the distinction between typical exercise discomfort and potential injury is crucial for your well-being.

There are lots of ways to learn about the best exercise techniques. Proper technique and form are very important when exercising, especially for women over 60. If you do exercises the wrong way, you could get hurt.

Exercising in front of a mirror lets you see if you're doing things correctly. It helps you keep an eye on your posture and movements to make sure they're on point. Besides, getting help from a certified trainer or physical therapist is a smart idea. They can show you the right way to do exercises and fix any mistakes you're making. If you can't meet them in person, you can check out online videos or virtual training sessions from trusted sources.

Some people prefer working out in a gym or at home with a friend, and others prefer exercising on their own. Whatever makes you feel most comfortable is the correct answer for yourself. Take your time to work through this book and ensure that you understand and feel comfortable with the information before starting your strength training journey.

12. Nutrition and Recovery

Importance of Proper Nutrition for Muscle Repair and Recovery

Muscle repair and recovery are fundamental components of any fitness or athletic program. The process of *muscle recovery* involves "repairing the muscle fibers that were broken down during exercise, replenishing energy stores, and removing waste products." Nutrition plays a pivotal role in these processes, influencing how effectively and quickly muscles can repair and grow stronger. This analysis delves into the importance of proper nutrition in muscle repair and recovery, examining the roles of macronutrients, micronutrients, hydration, timing, supplements, and specific dietary strategies for various populations (Mielgo-Ayuso & Fernández-Lázaro, 2021).

Understanding Muscle Repair and Recovery

Muscle repair and recovery involve a series of complex biological processes that begin as soon as exercise ends. When muscles are subjected to intense physical activity, especially resistance training, small tears occur in the muscle fibers. This microtrauma is a normal part of the muscle-building process (*How Microtears Help You*, n.d.).

During exercise, especially weight lifting or high-intensity interval training (HIIT), muscle fibers experience tiny tears. This causes an inflammatory response, leading to the delivery of blood and nutrients to the injured tissues. Subsequently, the body initiates the repair process. Satellite cells, a type of stem cell, become active and merge with the damaged muscle fibers to repair them, often resulting in their enlargement and increased strength (*How Microtears Help You*, n.d.).

Protein synthesis is the fundamental process by which cells construct proteins essential for repairing muscle tissues. Amino acids, the foundational elements of proteins, play a vital role in this mechanism. When protein is ingested, it breaks down into amino acids, which are then utilized for muscle tissue maintenance. To stimulate muscle growth and enhance recovery, the rate of protein synthesis should surpass that of protein breakdown. An optimal protein intake ensures a favorable protein equilibrium, supporting muscle repair and development (LaPelusa & Kaushik, 2022).

During muscle recovery, the intensity and type of exercise play major roles. High-intensity resistance training induces significant muscle damage, necessitating more extensive repair processes than low-intensity exercises. On the other hand, endurance exercises mainly deplete glycogen stores and cause minimal muscle damage, yet they still demand proper nutritional support for energy replenishment and repair of minor muscle damage (*High Intensity Exercise*, 2021).

Macronutrients and Muscle Recovery

Protein

High-quality protein sources encompass skinless poultry, low-fat dairy products, farm-fresh eggs, leguminous plants, and plant-derived proteins. Whey protein stands out for its rapid digestion and extensive amino acid profile, rendering it a favored option for recovery after physical exertion. Moreover, animal-based sources like chicken, beef, seafood, eggs, and dairy are regarded as complete proteins, boasting all essential amino acids. On the other hand, plant origins such as beans, lentils, quinoa, and tofu can be amalgamated to present a comprehensive amino acid array. Immediate protein intake within 30 minutes to 2 hours following a workout is crucial for optimizing muscle protein synthesis. Introducing protein before exercising can likewise diminish muscle degradation during physical activities (*Maximizing Muscle Recovery*, 2023).

Carbohydrates

Carbs are stored as glycogen in muscles and the liver. When you work out, glycogen stores get used up and need to be refilled for future workouts and to help with recovery. Whole grains, veggies, and legumes provide lasting energy, while fruits and dairy can quickly replenish glycogen. Having a mix of carbs and protein—usually in a 3:1 or 4:1 ratio—after exercising improves glycogen storage and muscle repair more effectively than just having protein alone (*Maximizing Muscle Recovery*, 2023).

Fats

Omega-3 and omega-6 fatty acids, known as healthy fats, play a vital role in reducing inflammation, supporting cell membrane health, and offering a sustained energy source. Sources rich in healthy fats include fatty fishlike salmon and mackerel, various nuts, seeds, avocados, and olive oil. It's important to exercise moderation when consuming fats around workout times to prevent slowdowns in digestion and nutrient absorption (*Maximizing Muscle Recovery*, 2023).

Micronutrients and Muscle Recovery

- *Vitamin D* is crucial for bone health and muscle function by enhancing calcium absorption, which is necessary for muscle contractions. Sources of vitamin D include sunlight, fortified foods, and supplements.
- *Vitamin C* is essential for collagen synthesis, aiding in the repair of connective tissues, and possesses antioxidant properties that reduce muscle damage. It can be found in citrus fruits, berries, and vegetables.
- *B complex* vitamins contribute to energy production and red blood cell formation, which is important for oxygen delivery to muscles during recovery. Sources of B complex vitamins include whole grains, meats, and leafy greens.
- *Calcium* is vital for muscle contraction and relaxation, preventing muscle cramps and spasms. It is found in dairy products, leafy greens, and fortified plant-based milks.
- *Magnesium* is involved in over 300 biochemical reactions, including protein synthesis and muscle function. Foods rich in magnesium are nuts, seeds, and whole grains.
- *Zinc* is essential for protein synthesis, cell growth, and immune function. Zinc sources include meat, shellfish, legumes, and seeds (Eastman, 2021).

Hydration and Muscle Recovery

Proper hydration is essential for maintaining optimal muscle function and preventing cramps. Water plays a key role in transporting nutrients to muscles and eliminating waste by-products. Adequate hydration supports blood volume, which is essential for supplying muscles with oxygen and nutrients during the recovery process.

Dehydration can result in decreased muscle strength and endurance, heightened injury susceptibility, and prolonged recovery periods. Even mild dehydration can hinder exercise performance and recovery efficiency. To ensure optimal hydration, it is recommended to consume water consistently leading up to exercise and to drink 16–20 oz of water 2–3 hours before working out. During exercise, aim to sip water regularly, targeting about 7–10 oz every 10–20 minutes. Following exercise, rehydrate by consuming water or electrolyte-rich beverages, particularly if you have perspired significantly. Strive to replenish lost fluids by ingesting 16–24 oz of water for every pound lost during exercise (Popkin et al., 2020).

Timing and Nutrient Intake

Prior to Exercising

- Carbohydrates are essential for stocking up on glycogen for energy before working out. Consume a well-rounded meal containing complex carbs and protein 2–3 hours before your session.
- Protein intake pre-workout aids in sustaining muscle protein levels and prevents excess breakdown during exercise.

- Ensure proper hydration prior to kick-starting your workout to maintain performance levels and stave off cramps.

During Exercise

- For extended or high-intensity sessions, consuming readily digestible carbohydrates can help maintain energy levels. Opt for sports drinks, gels, or fruits to fuel your body effectively.
- It's crucial to uphold the balance of electrolytes—sodium, potassium, and magnesium—during prolonged workouts, especially in hot climates.

Post-Workout Regimen

- Post-workout protein consumption is vital for muscle repair and growth. Target 20–40 g of top-notch protein within 30 minutes–2 hours after your workout.
- Replenish glycogen stores by consuming carbohydrates alongside protein. A carbohydrate-to-protein ratio of 3:1 or 4:1 is typically recommended for optimal recovery.
- While fat intake post-workout should be moderate to allow quick absorption of carbohydrates and proteins, incorporating healthy fats in meals later in the day can aid overall recovery and reduce inflammation (*Warm Up, Cool Down*, 2014).

Supplements for Muscle Recovery

Common Supplements

- *Protein powder,* known for its rapid absorption and provision of essential amino acids, is a preferred option for post-exercise recovery. Plant-based proteins such as pea, hemp, and soy serve as suitable alternatives for individuals with specific dietary requirements. This is extensively backed by research to facilitate muscle repair and growth under conditions of inadequate dietary protein intake. When consumed within recommended limits, the associated risks are minimal, although some individuals may experience digestive discomfort (*Health Benefits of Protein Powder*, 2018).
- *Branched-chain amino acids (BCAAs)* consist of leucine, isoleucine, and valine; they are vital amino acids that aid in alleviating muscle soreness and enhancing muscle protein synthesis. Existing evidence on their effectiveness is mixed; while certain studies demonstrate benefits in reducing soreness and muscle fatigue, others indicate that consuming complete protein sources might yield equally or more favorable results (*Benefits of Branched-Chain Amino Acid Supplements*, n.d.).
- *Creatine* functions by boosting muscle strength and power, enhancing high-intensity performance, and facilitating muscle recovery through the restoration of ATP reserves. Robust evidence underscores its role in enhancing muscle strength, power, and recovery. With general safety for most individuals, long-term usage warrants supervision concerning kidney function in susceptible cases (*Creatine*, 2023).

Guidelines for Supplement Use

- Consulting professionals: Always seek advice from a health care provider or nutritionist before initiating any new supplement, particularly if you have underlying health conditions. Emphasizing quality and dosage: Opt for high-quality, trusted brands, and adhere to recommended dosages. Remember, more is not necessarily better and may result in adverse effects at times.

Dietary Requirements Look Different for Us All

Older adults often need higher protein intake to counteract age-related muscle loss. Aim for 1.2–1.5 g of protein per kilogram of body weight. Focus on nutrient-rich, easily digestible foods to support muscle recovery without causing digestive discomfort. Include foods rich in calcium and vitamin D to support bone health, which is crucial for overall mobility and strength.

Individuals with specific dietary requirements, such as vegetarians and vegans, can fulfill their amino acid needs through plant-based sources like beans, lentils, tofu, tempeh, and quinoa. Ensuring a diverse intake of plant proteins will optimize amino acid intake. It's necessary to monitor levels of vital nutrients like vitamin B_{12}, iron, and zinc, which are required for muscle functionality and repair. Consider incorporating fortified foods or supplements for added support if needed (*Healthy Meal Planning*, n.d.).

Summary

Proper nutrition is vital for efficient muscle recovery. Understanding the significance of macronutrients, micronutrients, hydration, timing, and supplements allows individuals to optimize their dietary plans for improved recovery and enhanced performance. Embracing sound nutritional practices not only speeds up muscle recovery but also boosts overall well-being, minimizes injury risks, and underpins long-term fitness objectives. Adherence to these nutrition principles consistently promotes sustainable advancement and health. Whether you're an athlete, a senior citizen, or following specific dietary requirements, incorporating effective nutritional strategies is the cornerstone of reaching your fitness aspirations. With a tailored approach, you can bolster your body's recuperative mechanisms, develop stronger muscles, and enrich your lifestyle.

13. Hydration's Role in Strength Training

Proper hydration is a cornerstone of good health and overall well-being, playing a key role in various bodily functions. Individuals involved in strength training must pay special attention to maintaining adequate hydration levels as it significantly impacts their performance, recovery, and overall physical state. This examination explores the different facets of hydration concerning strength training, delving into the physiological mechanisms, the effects of dehydration, optimal hydration approaches, and specific considerations for diverse demographics.

Physiological Role of Hydration

Water plays a vital role in maintaining cellular equilibrium by supporting biochemical reactions, transporting nutrients, and removing waste from the body. It is necessary for preserving cell volume and integrity, which is particularly important for muscle cells during vigorous physical activity. Additionally, water aids in regulating body temperature through perspiration and respiration, thereby ensuring efficient cooling mechanisms, which are essential for preventing overheating during exercise. In addition, joint health and flexibility are supported by adequate hydration as water is a key component of synovial fluid, responsible for lubricating joints and minimizing injury risks during strength training.

Muscle Function and Hydration

Adequate water intake is essential for the proper functioning of muscles. It plays a major role in muscle contraction and relaxation by maintaining the balance of electrolytes necessary for the transmission of nerve signals that regulate muscle activity. Proper hydration is key in preventing muscle cramps and spasms, commonly triggered by imbalances in fluids and electrolytes. Moreover, hydration supports the transportation of nutrients to muscles and the expulsion of metabolic by-products, thereby promoting expedited recovery and muscle development.

Maintaining proper hydration is essential for efficient energy metabolism. Water is paramount for breaking down nutrients to generate ATP, the body's energy currency. Optimal hydration levels are key to supporting enduring performance throughout intense strength training sessions. Additionally, adequate hydration facilitates the elimination of metabolic by-products formed during physical activity, such as lactic acid, which is known to contribute to muscle fatigue and discomfort (*Water and Hydration*, n.d.).

EFFECTS OF DEHYDRATION ON STRENGTH TRAINING

Dehydration has a notable impact on muscle performance, leading to a significant decrease in muscle strength and power output. Even a slight level of dehydration, equivalent to one to two percent of body weight, can impede performance by reducing muscle function and coordination. Inadequate hydration expedites muscle fatigue, thereby curtailing the duration and intensity of strength training sessions. Consequently, this limitation hampers progress and diminishes the overall effectiveness of training endeavors.

Furthermore, dehydration has a negative impact on endurance and strength by hindering cardiovascular function and reducing blood volume. This leads to a decreased supply of oxygen and nutrients to muscles, posing challenges in maintaining prolonged physical exertion. Insufficient hydration also extends the recovery time by impeding the removal of metabolic waste products and compromising the effectiveness of nutrient transportation to muscles.

Moreover, dehydration significantly heightens the risk of muscle cramps, strains, and injuries by compromising muscle function and disrupting electrolyte balance. Prolonged dehydration can compromise joint and tendon health, rendering them more vulnerable to injuries during vigorous strength training sessions (*Water and Hydration*, n.d.).

OPTIMAL HYDRATION STRATEGIES FOR STRENGTH TRAINING

Water intake needs vary based on age, gender, weight, and activity level. A general recommendation is to consume 8–10 cups—2–2.5 L—of water daily, but individuals involved in athletics or strength training may require more hydration. Determine specific water requirements by considering body weight and physical activity, aiming for 0.5–1 oz of water per pound of body weight each day (Mayo Clinic Staff, 2020)

The Importance of Electrolytes

Electrolytes like sodium, potassium, calcium, and magnesium are vital for muscle function; they facilitate contractions and transmit nerve impulses. These essential minerals help regulate fluid balance inside and outside cells, which is key to sustaining optimal muscle performance and averting issues linked to dehydration (Shrimanker & Bhattarai, 2023).

Common Electrolytes

- Sodium is critical for regulating fluid balance and blood pressure. It is commonly found in table salt, sports drinks, and various food items.
- Potassium is essential for proper muscle function and transmitting nerve signals. Rich sources include bananas, potatoes, spinach, and oranges.
- Magnesium is vital for muscle contractions, promoting relaxation and aiding in protein synthesis. It can be sourced from nuts, seeds, whole grains, and leafy green vegetables.
- Calcium is crucial for muscle contractions and supporting overall bone health. Good sources include dairy products, fortified plant-based milks, and leafy green.

Enhancing Your Performance Through Electrolyte Balance

Optimize your performance by including electrolyte-rich foods in your diet. Choose from a variety of fruits, vegetables, nuts, seeds, and dairy products. For rapid replenishment of lost electrolytes and fluids post vigorous exercise, consider utilizing sports drinks (Shrimanker & Bhattarai, 2023).

Athletes have increased fluid requirements as they lose more sweat during intense training and competitions. Hence, tailor hydration plans according to individual sweat rates, exercise durations, and environmental factors to optimize performance.

As you age, your body may struggle to retain water and recognize thirst signals, leading to a higher risk of dehydration. It is essential to drink fluids regularly, even if you don't feel thirsty, and incorporate hydrating foods such as fruits and vegetables into your daily meals (Shrimanker & Bhattarai, 2023).

Individuals managing conditions like diabetes or kidney disease may have distinct hydration requirements, necessitating tailored guidance from health care professionals. Besides, certain medications can influence hydration levels, prompting the need for adjustments in fluid consumption. Thus, it is essential to seek advice from your health care provider for personalized recommendations, (Bonvissuto, 2018).

Hydration and Nutrient Absorption

Staying properly hydrated impacts your body's ability to absorb nutrients efficiently. Adequate hydration ensures swift transport of nutrients to muscles and tissues, bolstering overall health and performance. Water is key in aiding the digestion and absorption of nutrients, enhancing their availability for muscle recovery and repair. It also plays a crucial role in the interaction with vitamins and minerals. Water-soluble vitamins such as B complex and C rely on adequate hydration for optimal absorption and utilization in the body. Essential electrolytes like sodium, potassium, calcium, and magnesium also necessitate sufficient water for efficient transport and absorption into the body. Maintaining proper hydration levels supports the equilibrium of these vital minerals, contributing to enhanced muscle functionality and faster recovery processes (*The Contribution of Drinking Water*, 1980).

Hydration and Protein Synthesis

Water helps break down and absorb proteins and amino acids. Proper hydration is essential for optimal digestive system function, ensuring efficient nutrient uptake. In addition, it aids in muscle protein synthesis by enabling the transportation of amino acids to muscle tissues. Sufficient water intake is vital for maintaining the cellular environment needed for muscle repair and growth (Waldegger et al., 1997).

There are many misconceptions when it comes to hydration. One misconception is that waiting until you're thirsty to drink water is enough. However, thirst doesn't always signal proper hydration; it could mean you're already somewhat dehydrated. Hence, it's crucial to regularly consume water throughout the day. Another myth suggests that dark urine always means dehydration. While it can indicate dehydration, certain foods, medicines, or supplements can also darken urine. Consistently monitoring urine color and frequency is a better way to assess hydration levels. Lastly, the belief that sports drinks are vital for everyone is not accurate. For most individuals, especially those in moderate physical activity, water suffices for hydration. Sports drinks only become beneficial during intense, prolonged workout sessions, leading to substantial electrolyte loss (*Water and Hydration*, n.d.).

Considerations for proper hydration include individual variations in needs, influenced by factors like age, weight, activity levels, and environmental circumstances. Developing personalized hydration plans is essential. Note that overconsumption of water may result in hyponatremia, a serious condition characterized by dangerously low blood sodium levels. Hence, achieving a harmonious equilibrium is pivotal for maintaining optimal hydration levels.

Track your daily water intake by monitoring the amount you drink. Utilize a water bottle with measurements to track your consumption. In addition, enhance your hydration by incorporating water-rich foods such as fruits, vegetables, and soups into your diet. Set reminders using alarms or apps to ensure consistent water consumption, especially if you lead a hectic life or have a tendency to forget.

Proper hydration offers numerous long-term benefits by supporting muscle health, enhancing performance, and promoting overall well-being. It plays a vital role in preventing chronic conditions, boosting cognitive function, and facilitating metabolic processes.

Hydration stands as a key element in every strength training routine. Prioritizing sufficient fluid intake and employing effective hydration methods can help individuals optimize training capabilities, hasten recovery, and sustain their well-being. Whether you are an experienced athlete, an aging individual, or embarking on a fitness journey, understanding and practicing adequate hydration is essential for accomplishing strength training objectives and leading a healthier life.

14. Overcoming Challenges and Staying Motivated

Dealing With Age-Related Health Issues and Chronic Conditions

Following a health-conscious lifestyle is crucial for overall well-being; however, the interplay of genetics, age, and daily habits, influences our susceptibility to developing chronic health conditions. While preventive measures can mitigate health issues to some extent, complete avoidance is unattainable. As we read in Chapter 2, we know that strength training is so much more than being able to carry your own bags or getting up from the couch by yourself. Exercising, specifically strength training, is imperative for a healthier and longer life.

Incorporating strength training into your routine may present challenges, especially as you age and confront new health concerns or chronic illnesses. Embracing strength training demands innovation and perseverance, even during times when progress seems stagnant. Always consult health care providers before attempting any exercises, as they can provide guidance on safe practices and necessary modifications.

This guide delves into various modifications and movement patterns. The diversity of strength exercises offers ample options to design your own personalized workout routine. Embrace each effort as part of your journey and avoid viewing the inability to complete a movement as a setback; there are many agile, fit, young, and healthy people unable to do certain exercises! Prioritize your well-being and listen to your body; there will be days when you feel less than optimal. Adjust your pace, reduce repetitions, or skip a workout if needed, ensuring your exercise routine enhances rather than harms your health. Maintaining consistent motivation is necessary, especially when managing chronic or intermittent illnesses that disrupt your routine. Remember, the absence of physical activity can exacerbate existing health conditions or lead to new ones.

Helpful Tips

- Set clear objectives as constant reminders of your purpose.
- Establish a consistent schedule by allocating specific times for strength training, allowing mental readiness and logistical organization.
- Arrange your environment and tools to adhere consistently to this schedule.
- Monitoring your advancements can serve as a potent motivator, commemorating achievements such as enhanced strength or stamina.
- Design your workout routine to be enjoyable, seamlessly integrating it into your daily life by exploring various exercises and adjustments.

- Recognize that adjustments are tailored for specific needs or constraints. If a certain exercise presents difficulties, consider adapted versions or alternative moves, like utilizing resistance bands or exploring aqua-based workouts.
- Finally, prioritize self-nurturing by recognizing the significance of rest and being attuned to your body's cues while consulting with medical professionals.

It is very important that you do not hurt yourself. Some days, you might feel a bit under the weather or not up to a big workout, this is completely normal! On these days, move slower, do fewer repetitions of exercises, or skip working out, but most importantly, listen to your body! Exercise is supposed to make you feel good and not injure you.

Staying motivated can be quite difficult, especially if you live with a chronic, long-term, or intermittent illness, as it throws off your routine; however, it is important to note that not exercising at all can worsen many illnesses or create new health issues. Thus, you must follow a few strategies to help you stay committed to your fitness goals.

First, set clear goals. Once you have short- and long-term goals written down, they will be constant reminders as to why you are doing what you are doing. Consistency is key! Create a routine where you specifically set out times in the week for your strength training. Planning it gives you the opportunity to mentally prepare yourself, arrange your trip to the gym, or prep your home space for the training. It is easier to get into a workout routine if you have all the necessary things organized.

Tracking your progress can also be a wonderful tool. It feels amazing when you are able to lift a bag that would usually hurt too much. You feel elated at your ability to walk faster or further without the need for assistance. Thus, tracking the number of repetitions of the exercises you completed in each training session will be motivating.

Being able to look at yourself growing stronger is a unique and wonderful experience, and making your exercise routine enjoyable is of utmost importance. Remember, it is not supposed to be torturous to exercise; it is part of your lifestyle. Play around with different exercises and their modifications.

It is important to note that exercise modifications are there for a reason; if you struggle to complete a specific exercise, there is either an adapted version available or a similar exercise that can be done. Adaptions can range from using resistance bands instead of weights to water-based exercises.

Above all else, remember that it is completely fine if you need to slow down or take a few days off. Listening to your body and your health care provider is, first and foremost, important.

FINDING SUPPORT FROM PEERS, TRAINERS, AND ONLINE COMMUNITIES

Sharing your journey with others is not necessary, but it can be beneficial. It is sometimes very difficult to find motivation when you feel depressed or struggling to integrate the correct exercises into your lifestyle. Having supportive friends, family, and, in some cases, a professional trainer can help you get started, stay strong, and grow in your new journey. It is also important to note that in some cases, support might not be available from friends and family. People differ, and this is an unfortunate reality that cannot be controlled. In this context, it is important to remember that there are wonderful online groups of people going through a similar journey to yours. Talking to people at different points in their journey can give you a glimpse of what to expect in a few weeks or a few years, and you will also be able to support others by sharing your own experience!

Positivity is the key. While it is healthy and important to address the difficulties, it is essential to surround yourself with people who will validate how you feel and not pull you deeper down into negative feelings.

There are many different ways to gain a supportive group of peers. Join a fitness class (e.g., aerobics, water aerobics, yoga, strength training group, etc.), whether online or in person. The group setting and safe environment will provide you with a sense of camaraderie rarely found elsewhere. Joining a neighborhood exercise group or a community center will also provide a safe space.

Working alongside a skilled personal trainer can vastly impact the success of a strength training regimen tailored for women aged 60 and above. These professionals offer individualized direction, ensure exercises are executed accurately, and adapt routines to suit specific needs and objectives. When selecting a trainer, seek out those with a proven track record in assisting older individuals and a deep understanding of age-related health concerns. Acquiring certifications from esteemed bodies like the National Academy of Sports Medicine (NASM) or the American Council on Exercise (ACE) serves as a reliable gauge of a trainer's expertise. Through personalized training plans, personal trainers can craft specialized strength training regimens that consider unique fitness levels, health conditions, and aspirations. This bespoke approach not only fosters safety but also maximizes effectiveness.

Trainers oversee progress closely and tweak training plans as necessary, with regular check-ins playing a major role in maintaining motivation and achieving set goals. Beyond facilitating workouts, trainers offer invaluable insights into the significance of strength training, proper nutrition, and other facets of a wholesome lifestyle. Embracing this comprehensive methodology can bolster overall well-being and pave the way for enduring success. For those inclined to work out from home or lacking access to local trainers, virtual training sessions conducted via video calls emerge as a viable alternative. Numerous trainers extend online services, delivering the same caliber of support and guidance as in-person sessions.

In the digital age, accessing support and resources for strength training has become more convenient than ever for women over 60. Online communities, forums, and fitness platforms cater to this demographic by providing a plethora of information and fostering a sense of camaraderie. Various websites and apps offer strength training programs tailored for older adults, complete with video tutorials, workout plans, and tools for tracking progress.

Moreover, engaging in fitness-related discussions on platforms like Reddit, MyFitnessPal, and health forums allows users to share experiences, seek advice, and gain valuable insights. Additionally, YouTube channels hosted by fitness experts and trainers offer free workout videos and tutorials, serving as an excellent resource for learning new exercises and maintaining motivation. For individuals seeking more comprehensive knowledge, platforms also offer online courses and webinars on fitness and health topics, providing practical tips for strength training. In addition, fitness apps such as FitOn and SilverSneakers GO deliver customized workout programs, tracking capabilities, and virtual classes, offering a convenient way to receive continued guidance and support.

Strength training offers numerous benefits for women over 60, enhancing physical health, mental well-being, and overall quality of life. Obstacles like age-related health issues and chronic conditions can be overcome. Besides, embracing strength training, with support from peers, trainers, and online communities, allows women to enjoy its advantages. Furthermore, motivation and consistency are vital for long-term success in strength training. Setting clear goals, establishing a routine, tracking progress, engaging in enjoyable activities, seeking support, and staying informed contribute to an effective fitness regimen. Leveraging support systems helps women over 60 navigate challenges and lead stronger, healthier, and more active lives in their golden years.

Setting Realistic Expectations and Celebrating Progress

While the advantages of strength training are indisputable, it is crucial for women in their sixties to have reasonable expectations when commencing a strength training regimen to avoid discouragement and maintain motivation.

To set achievable objectives effectively, it is essential to start gradually by establishing a manageable routine, particularly for novices in strength training. Initiate with lighter weights and progressively elevate the intensity to prevent injuries and nurture self-assurance. Define specific and measurable goals rather than vague aims like merely *getting stronger*. For instance, aim for specifics such as *increasing lifting capacity by 10 lbs within 3 months* or *performing 15 squats unaided*.

Consistency is paramount for progress; hence, prioritizing regular, albeit brief, strength training sessions is more fruitful than sporadic, prolonged workouts. Attune to your body's responses during exercise; while mild muscle soreness is typical, acute pain or discomfort signals the need to discontinue and seek professional advice.

In this setting, customizing exercises to accommodate preexisting health conditions or physical constraints ensures safety and efficacy, with input from a health care provider or fitness expert offering valuable direction. Patience is fundamental, as results may unfold gradually, particularly in the initial phases of building strength and muscle; acknowledging and celebrating incremental advancements along the journey is key to sustaining motivation and progress.

To maintain motivation and commitment to a strength training program, it is crucial to celebrate progress effectively. Building confidence through acknowledging even the smallest achievements can inspire ongoing dedication. Optimal strategies for recognizing progress include tracking your development in a workout journal to visually witness improvement, breaking down larger objectives into manageable milestones, rewarding yourself upon goal achievement, reflecting on non-scale victories such as enhanced energy levels and mood, monitoring visual progress through regular photos, and engaging with a fitness support group for collective motivation and camaraderie. Celebrating advancements in fitness goes beyond physical outcomes and serves as a significant factor in sustaining enthusiasm and progress.

To ensure sustained success, establish a strength training regimen that is enduring and engaging. Essential tips to craft an effective routine include the following points:

- Prioritize workouts: Approach your workouts with a commitment level akin to scheduled appointments.

Consistent effort is paramount for witnessing tangible progress.

- Embrace variety: Infuse your routine with diverse exercises, equipment, and workout styles to maintain interest and target varying muscle groups.
- Listen to your body: Monitoring your body's responses is crucial; make necessary adjustments to your regimen. Recognize that sufficient rest and recovery are as imperative as the workouts themselves.
- Stay educated: Continuously enhance your knowledge of strength training methodologies, nutritional aspects, and overall wellness. Being well-informed facilitates better decision-making and sustains motivation.
- Cultivate enjoyment: Opt for activities and exercises that bring you genuine pleasure. Finding fulfillment in your workouts increases the likelihood of prolonged commitment.

Strength training is a vital tool for women aged 60 and above to improve physical health, mental well-being, and overall quality of life. Setting achievable goals and acknowledging progress fuel motivation and aid in reaching fitness targets. This type of exercise helps maintain muscle mass, enhance bone density, improve balance, increase metabolism, and support mental wellness.

Overcoming obstacles, focusing on nutrition, and establishing a consistent routine are key factors for long-term success. Adopting strength training with a strategic approach can result in a more resilient, healthier, and satisfying lifestyle during one's later years.

15. Long-Term Maintenance and Sustainability

As you age, maintaining your strength and bodily functions becomes increasingly vital. Strength training enhances your physical health and overall quality of life. It also preserves your independence and, thus, your lifestyle. The key is to remember that the benefits lie in your ability to sustain your strength training journey in the long term.

There are various strategies to ensure the long-term sustainability and maintenance of your strength training journey.

Setting Realistic and Achievable Goals

We discussed setting realistic and achievable goals in Chapter 7. It is imperative that you set short-term and long-term goals, as this is what will help you through the difficult days. Your short-term goals will stay in the forefront of your mind, a target close by that will help you keep your momentum. The results of your short-term goals are small, whereas long-term goals provide a broader view, and accomplishing these goals will take some time. Your short-term goals should eventually lead you to your long-term goals.

Creating a Sustainable Routine

Feeling frustrated and impatient at the slow-moving progress in the initial stages of your workout routine is a common experience. Rushing the process can be counterproductive, potentially pushing your body beyond its limits. Consistency is key for sustainable results, ensuring long-term benefits. Besides, flexibility in your routine is essential, allowing adjustments for unexpected events like vacations without compromising progress. Skipping a session occasionally or rescheduling is understandable if it clashes with an event. Your workout routine is there to improve your lifestyle, not replace it!

Incorporating Recovery and Rest

This further explains the importance of sustaining your routine; pushing yourself too far past your limitations without sufficiently resting can be very detrimental. Rest is essential for your muscles to recover and ensure that you do not injure yourself and that muscle repair and growth—which is the whole reason we are doing these exercises—can take place. It is important to have a rest day scheduled in your week—maybe you take a walk or do yoga during these days. Overall, it is important that you listen to your body and learn to recognize the difference between normal soreness from completing a good exercise and pain from overexertion or injury.

Maintaining Motivation

One of the best ways to maintain motivation over the long term is by keeping a workout journal. We spoke about this in Chapter 6. Redoing the initial assessments after a few months on your workout regime can be very motivating. It provides you with a clear view of just how much you have improved, even if it does not necessarily feel like you did. We also discussed in Chapter 14 the importance of having a supportive system. Being able to share your difficulties as well as your achievements makes you feel connected and motivated.

Adapting to Changes

Adjust the workout routine as physical abilities and life circumstances evolve. This involves modifying exercise intensity, incorporating diverse equipment, and adjusting workout frequency. Embrace adaptability to maintain a safe, effective, and personalized strength training regimen aligned with current requirements.

Continually educating oneself about proper techniques and new exercises is key to maintaining a safe and effective strength training routine. Utilizing resources such as instructional videos, books, and professional trainers can enhance understanding and execution. Continuous learning keeps the routine fresh and helps prevent the onset of injury through proper form and technique.

Education and Resources

It is important to remember that as time goes on, more research is done, new information is regularly released, and new exercises are made available regularly.

Educating yourself in regards to the proper manner to complete exercises, as well as on the development of new—and possibly more efficient—exercises, is imperative. Many resources are available, such as educational videos, books, booklets, articles, or trained professionals. Using these resources will ensure that you are as informed as possible. It is important to adjust your routine from time to time to ensure that you do not get bored or overexert certain muscles.

Safety Considerations

Safety should be the top priority. To prevent injuries, it's necessary to maintain proper form, use the right equipment, and include warm-up and cooldown routines. When beginning a fitness journey, working with a certified trainer is essential for personalized guidance and ensuring the correct execution of exercises.

Balanced Nutrition

Nutrition is pivotal in supporting the endeavors of strength training. Ample protein intake is required for the repair and growth of muscles while maintaining hydration boosts overall exercise performance and aids in recovery. A well-rounded diet abundant in fruits, vegetables, whole grains, and healthy fats supplies the essential nutrients required for sustained energy levels and promoting optimal health.

Mind-Body Connection

Practicing mindfulness through meditation or deep breathing can boost mental well-being and alleviate stress. Engaging in yoga not only enhances flexibility and joint health but also nurtures a profound mind-body harmony, supporting overall health.

Routine Health Checks

Regular visits to health care providers assist in monitoring health conditions and maintaining the safety and effectiveness of the exercise regimen. Evaluations of bone density and muscle mass at intervals can offer valuable insights into the strength training program's efficacy and inform any required modifications.

Social and Community Engagement

Participating in group fitness classes or community events fosters social interaction and offers a supportive setting for sustaining a fitness regimen. Social bonds boost motivation and responsibility, facilitating adherence to the regimen.

Technology and Gadgets

Utilizing fitness monitoring devices and applications can offer in-depth insights into activity levels and progress and pinpoint areas for enhancement. Online platforms that provide workout tutorials and virtual coaching sessions simplify the process of staying physically active at home, granting flexibility and convenience.

Improving the quality of life and preserving independence for women aged 60 and above hinges on consistent engagement in strength training. Setting realistic goals, establishing a sustainable routine, prioritizing adequate recovery, and persisting with motivation are essential elements for ensuring the durability of their strength training program. Furthermore, integrating strength training into a well-rounded lifestyle encompassing balanced nutrition, mindfulness practices, routine health screenings, and active social participation contributes significantly to overall well-being. With unwavering commitment and effective strategies, strength training can evolve into a rewarding and enduring part of daily life, fostering health and vitality well into the senior years.

ADAPTING WORKOUTS TO CHANGING NEEDS AND ABILITIES

Nothing in life stays the same; as time goes on, our bodies change as well. Our physical capabilities and health conditions naturally change. This does mean we must adjust our workouts to meet our changing abilities and needs. As we discussed, strength training is exceptionally important to combat muscle mass and muscle strength loss as well as loss of bone density. This does not stop us from aging though, and we must adjust the types of exercises we do to take these changes into consideration. This will ensure the training is effective, safe, and enjoyable.

As humans age, their bodies undergo distinct physiological changes. These changes encompass a natural decrease in muscle mass and bone density, reduced flexibility in joints, longer recovery periods, and an elevated vulnerability to injuries. Moreover, conditions like arthritis, osteoporosis, and cardiovascular ailments may surface or progress, further impacting physical capabilities. The initial step toward adapting strength training regimens to sustain health and fitness objectives without causing harm involves acknowledging these alterations (Volpi et al., 2004).

Personalized workouts start by considering an individual's fitness level, health status, and physical limitations. Assessments, possibly overseen by a fitness expert or health care professional, offer valuable insights for adjusting exercises. Managing the principle of progressive overload involves gradually intensifying exercise duration, complexity, and intensity to match evolving abilities.

Joint health is essential as we age, especially for individuals dealing with conditions like arthritis. Modifying exercise routines to incorporate joint-friendly movements can ease discomfort and lower the chance of injuries. This adjustment could mean swapping high-impact activities with gentler options, such as choosing an elliptical machine over running or engaging in water-based workouts that lessen joint strain. Including exercises that boost joint flexibility and stability, like yoga and Pilates, can also enhance a strength training plan. Additionally, functional fitness activities that mimic daily actions can enhance the overall quality of life by improving the capacity to handle everyday responsibilities and focusing on enhancing coordination, balance, and mobility, which are essential to maintaining independence. Integrating strength training with functional movements, such as squats, lunges, and step-ups, can assist women aged 60 and above in preserving functional abilities and reducing the likelihood of falls and injuries.

As flexibility tends to decrease with age, it is essential to incorporate flexibility and mobility exercises into a strength training regimen. Including stretching exercises, dynamic warm-ups, and activities such as yoga can aid in preserving and enhancing flexibility, alleviating stiffness, and boosting overall movement quality. This harmonious blend of strength and flexibility not only enhances performance in strength training routines but also fosters an increased range of motion and lowers the likelihood of injuries.

If you feel unsure, seek guidance from experienced fitness professionals specialized in working with older adults when adapting strength training routines. These experts offer personalized recommendations, guaranteeing proper form and designing comprehensive workout plans that target strength, flexibility, endurance, and functional fitness.

By personalizing and progressively adjusting exercises, emphasizing joint-friendly movements, incorporating functional fitness, balancing strength with flexibility, and listening to the body, women can continue to reap the benefits of strength training safely and effectively. Moreover, leveraging professional guidance and embracing a holistic approach to fitness ensures that strength training remains a rewarding and sustainable part of a healthy lifestyle, supporting vitality and independence well into the later years.

Listen to your body during workouts. Pain, extreme fatigue, or prolonged recovery times signal the need for adjustments. Modify or skip uncomfortable exercises to prioritize safety and efficacy in your fitness routine. Adapting workouts means taking a comprehensive approach to health and fitness. This involves maintaining a balanced diet that supports muscle health, staying hydrated, ensuring adequate sleep, and managing stress levels. Furthermore, including activities like meditation and social interactions that enhance mental well-being can improve the efficiency and sustainability of your fitness routine.

CULTIVATING A LIFELONG COMMITMENT TO HEALTH AND FITNESS

Commencing a journey of strength training and overall fitness can be life-changing at any age. However, for women over 60, it offers distinct advantages that extend well beyond physical prowess. The focus lies in nurturing a lifelong dedication to health and well-being that can elevate quality of life, enhance longevity, and infuse daily living with happiness.

Regular exercise not only releases endorphins to alleviate symptoms of depression and anxiety but also boosts cognitive function and delays the onset of dementia. In addition, participating in fitness classes or groups can foster new friendships and essential social support networks that significantly impact mental health (Volpi et al., 2004).

Setting goals is important and very helpful:

1. Start with easily attainable objectives, such as committing to a brief 15-minute daily walk and participating in a weekly yoga session.
2. Progress gradually by increasing the intensity and duration of your exercise routines.
3. Celebrate minor achievements to maintain motivation.
4. Collaborate with a fitness expert to develop a customized program that suits your individual needs and capabilities. This guarantees a safe and efficient fitness regimen.

To ensure success in your fitness journey, establishing and adhering to a consistent workout schedule is paramount. Consistency not only aids in habit formation but also simplifies adherence to your fitness regimen. Embrace variety in your exercises by incorporating a diverse range of workout modalities such as strength training, cardiovascular activities, flexibility drills, and exercises that enhance balance.

Engage in activities you genuinely love, such as dancing, swimming, hiking, or gardening, to find joy. Practices like yoga and tai chi enhance both physical strength and the profound connection between mind and body, ultimately boosting overall well-being.

Socialize with like-minded individuals by becoming part of local or online fitness groups. These communities offer encouragement, accountability, and a sense of companionship to boost your fitness journey. In addition, enlist the support of family and friends in your fitness endeavors. Share your progress and goals with them, encouraging joint exercise sessions or leveraging their backing for additional motivation.

Embrace a holistic approach! To cultivate a lifelong commitment to health and fitness, you must do more than a strength training regime. You must adjust your nutritional intake, focusing on a balanced diet rich in nutrients. Proper nutrition, with a healthy amount of protein, supports muscle repair and overall health. As important as it is to exercise and eat healthy, it is just as important to rest and recover. Get an adequate amount of sleep every night and take some time to relax to ensure your body has enough time to recover, which helps maintain energy levels and prevent injuries.

Maintaining a lifelong dedication to health and fitness proves to be a rewarding pursuit that elevates every facet of life. Women aged 60 and above can significantly boost their physical health, mental acuity, and emotional wellness through strength training and consistent exercise. By establishing achievable objectives, exploring enjoyable physical activities, garnering support, and embracing a comprehensive approach, one can initiate a lasting fitness journey that ignites happiness and vigor for years ahead. Remember, commencing at any age is opportune, and each incremental progress marks a triumph in itself.

16. Incorporating Cardiovascular and Flexibility Exercises for Overall Fitness

This book specifically focuses on strength training, understanding its importance, as well as how to implement it into your life. This does not mean that this is the only form of exercise that your body needs. On the contrary, your body requires a variety of different exercises. Here, we will lightly touch on the importance of cardio and flexibility exercises as well as provide you with a few options to integrate into your exercise routine.

Make sure you engage in exercises that correspond to your current fitness level and overall health. If you're a beginner or have health concerns, it's advisable to initiate with gentle and less demanding exercises. Progress as you improve by gradually increasing the duration or intensity of your workout regimen. Moreover, prioritize safety during your workout sessions. Proper execution of exercises ensures your safety and maximizes their effectiveness. If unsure about the suitability of an exercise, seek guidance from a fitness professional or consult with a health care provider.

Everyone should engage in cardiovascular activities such as walking, swimming, cycling, and dancing to maintain their heart's health and strength. These activities strengthen the heart muscle, promote better blood circulation, and may reduce blood pressure. Engaging in such physical activities can also contribute to increased vitality and happiness. Opting for brisk walking, swimming, or cycling can intensify the heart's workload, benefiting overall health. Moreover, dancing is an enjoyable way to stay active and maintain heart health. It's essential to exercise at a challenging yet manageable intensity level without overexerting yourself. Aim for a minimum of 30 minutes of daily exercise for 5 days each week, starting at a comfortable pace and gradually increasing intensity as your fitness improves.

Regular cardiovascular exercise is essential for heart health, increased lung capacity, and enhanced overall stamina. Engaging in consistent cardio activities aids in weight management, reduces the risk of chronic conditions, and promotes mental well-being.

In general, engaging in physical activity strengthens the heart and enhances circulation, thereby reducing the likelihood of heart disease and stroke. Physical exercise aids in burning calories and supporting weight maintenance, thus contributing to overall well-being. Furthermore, it triggers the release of endorphins that elevate mood and energy levels. Consistent exercise is associated with a reduced risk of chronic ailments such as diabetes, high blood pressure, and certain types of cancer (Nystoriak & Bhatnagar, 2018).

Incorporating Cardio exercises into your routine is vital for overall health. Walking, a gentle yet effective form of cardio, can be easily integrated into your daily life with a goal of 30 minutes most days. Swimming offers a full-body workout without impacting the joints, making it ideal for those with joint concerns.

Cycling, whether indoor or outdoor, is a versatile option that boosts cardiovascular fitness and can be tailored to different intensity levels. Dancing is not only a joyful way to elevate your heart rate but also an opportunity to revel in music and movement. For a more interactive experience, consider engaging in group classes such as aerobics, Zumba, or water aerobics, which provide not only the physical benefits of cardio but also the social and motivational support that comes with a group setting (Nystoriak & Bhatnagar, 2018).

Flexibility exercises benefit women over 60 by improving joint mobility, enhancing balance and posture, and reducing tension. This regimen holds particular significance for older adults as it plays a crucial role in preserving their ability to move freely and live independently. Incorporating stretching into your routine promotes muscle relaxation and overall well-being. Practices like yoga, Pilates, or tai chi help strengthen the body and enhance flexibility, balance, and mental acuity, which are particularly beneficial for older individuals.

Regular stretching offers a plethora of benefits for overall well-being. It enhances mobility by maintaining joint flexibility, which is crucial for daily functions. Moreover, it aids in injury prevention by keeping muscles supple, decreasing the chances of strains and sprains. Stretching also plays a vital role in pain reduction, particularly in alleviating discomfort associated with conditions such as arthritis by combating stiffness. Additionally, it contributes to improved posture and balance, subsequently lowering the likelihood of falls.

Regular stretching sessions several times a week maintain body flexibility and functionality. Including these exercises before and after your workouts aids in warming up and cooling down your muscles effectively. It is necessary to perform these exercises mindfully to prevent injury, seeking guidance from a medical professional or fitness instructor if needed.

Incorporating Flexibility Exercises Into Your Routine

Incorporating flexibility into your daily routine can bring numerous benefits. You can start by including stretching exercises focusing on major muscle groups, holding each stretch for 15–30 seconds, and repeating 2–4 times. Additionally, practicing yoga, a holistic discipline that integrates flexibility, strength, and balance, can be fruitful, especially if you opt for classes specifically designed for seniors or beginners. Tai chi, a gentle form of martial arts characterized by its flowing movements, is renowned for enhancing flexibility and balance and promoting mental relaxation, while Pilates is another excellent option that emphasizes core strength, flexibility, and overall body awareness, with many exercises easily adaptable to different fitness levels (*Stretching*, 2022).

CREATING A BALANCED ROUTINE

A well-rounded weekly exercise routine should consist of various components to promote overall fitness and well-being. Cardiovascular exercise is essential for heart health, with a recommended minimum of 150 minutes per week of moderate-intensity cardio, achievable through daily 30-minute sessions. In addition, incorporating flexibility exercises 2–3 times weekly, with daily stretching after workouts, helps maintain mobility and prevent injury. Strength training is crucial for muscle development and should target all major muscle groups 2–3 times a week. To optimize your workout, include warm-up and cooldown sessions to prepare your body and aid recovery. On rest days, engage in light activities to keep your body active without straining it. Note that listening to your body's signals is vital; adjust workout intensity accordingly and prioritize rest and recovery to prevent overexertion and promote muscle repair and growth.

Summary

Incorporating cardiovascular and flexibility workouts into your exercise regimen is necessary for maintaining overall health and well-being, particularly for women aged 60 and above. These exercises not only enhance strength training but also offer distinct advantages that boost heart health, flexibility, and mental acuity. By establishing a well-rounded and enjoyable fitness routine, you can uphold an active lifestyle that aligns with your objectives and enhances your quality of life. Remember, maintaining regularity and attuning to your body's needs is fundamental for sustaining a successful fitness journey.

Conclusion

Recap of Key Takeaways and Insights

Strength training requires diligent preparation and planning for safe and successful outcomes. Emphasizing the significance of initiating strength training, the commitment of time and effort yields invaluable returns. While embarking on this journey may appear daunting for women above 60, the resulting strength and autonomy gained from adhering to a training regimen make it truly rewarding.

After reading this book, you are now equipped with the necessary knowledge, tools, and encouragement needed to confidently and securely embrace strength training. By integrating this practice into your routine, you are making a lasting investment in your physical wellness, mental health, and overall longevity. The benefits of strength training are vast, ranging from increased muscle mass and bone density to enhanced balance and cognitive function, enabling you to sustain independence, engage in daily activities, and pursue a fulfilling life.

A few key takeaways to remember

1. Start slow and progress gradually: After assessing your fitness levels, you have a very good idea of your current physical abilities. Set up your workout regime in a way that you will be able to complete it. As time goes on and you become stronger, gradually increase the exercises. Consistency and patience are crucial for long-term success.

2. Listen to your body: Pay attention to how your body responds to different exercises. While exercising pushes you to become stronger, it is still supposed to be enjoyable and not excruciating to complete. If you need to remove an exercise and replace it with one that is less painful, do so. Most important of all, rest and recovery are as necessary as the workouts themselves. Your muscles need time off to repair for the next workout.

3. Balance and variety: Incorporate a mix of strength training, cardiovascular exercise, flexibility, and balance workouts because not one or the other is sufficient. Your body needs cardio workouts for one reason, strength training for another, etc. By incorporating the different types of exercises, you ensure a well-rounded fitness regimen.

4. Seek support and stay motivated: If you prefer to have your fitness journey as something private, that is completely fine! It is important to remember that our supportive communities provide us with immense power. Whether it's sharing your journey with a single friend, your partner, or an in-person or online fitness community, having support can significantly help you stay motivated. If you are worried about receiving unsolicited comments from others, set boundaries!

Learning to set healthy boundaries is a journey on its own.

5. Celebrate your progress: Acknowledge and celebrate your achievements, no matter how small. Each step forward is a victory on your path to better health. We all progress at different paces, and it is important not to compare yourself with others but to focus on your own journey and accomplishments.

Remember, strength training is not just about lifting weights; it's about lifting your spirits, enhancing your health, and embracing a vibrant and active lifestyle. You have the power to shape your future, and by committing to strength training, you are taking a proactive step toward a healthier, stronger, and more fulfilling life.

Your journey is unique, and so are your goals and challenges. Be kind to yourself, enjoy the process, and keep pushing forward. The benefits of strength training extend far beyond the gym—they enrich every aspect of your life. With determination and the right approach, you can continue to grow stronger, more resilient, and more confident every day.

Here's to your strength, health, and unwavering spirit. Keep moving, keep challenging yourself, and most importantly, keep believing in your incredible potential. The best is yet to come.

ENCOURAGEMENT TO CONTINUE ON THE JOURNEY TO AGING STRONG

Embarking on a strength training journey is an empowering step toward maintaining health and vitality, especially for women over 60. The preparation before starting the journey might seem daunting, but actually, starting the exercise routine and sticking to it are even more difficult to face. This is not a diet that you follow for a few weeks until you have lost weight and then go back to your old unsustainable eating habits. This is a lifestyle change, a lifelong commitment. As you progress, it's essential to stay motivated and encouraged, reminding yourself of the benefits of your commitment.

Here are a few things that you can remind yourself of if you waver during your journey:

- Recognize your achievements: Celebrate milestones by recognizing your achievements in your fitness journey. Every new weight lifted, additional rep, or improvement in form deserves applause. Take a moment to reflect on the distance you've covered since you began this journey. These achievements showcase your unwavering dedication and effort. To stay motivated, consider tracking your progress. Whether through a fitness journal or workout app, observing your advancements in writing supports the positive transformations occurring within your body.
- Embrace the benefits: Embracing the benefits of physical strength offers multiple advantages. Building muscle not only makes everyday tasks easier, such as carrying groceries or playing with grandchildren, but also enhances your overall quality of life. Engaging in strength training is vital for bone health, as it helps combat osteoporosis by increasing bone density and lowering the risk of fractures, especially as you age and your bones become more fragile. Additionally, regular exercise, including strength training, releases endorphins, the body's natural mood enhancers, which can alleviate symptoms of depression and anxiety, promoting a more positive perspective on life. Moreover, the maintenance of strength and mobility promotes independence, allowing individuals to stay self-reliant for

a longer time and partake in activities they love without depending on others.

Inspirational stories: Draw inspiration from other women who have taken up strength training later in life as role models. Their experiences can serve as motivation, reinforcing the idea that commencing and thriving in strength training know no age limit. Consider your personal journey as well. What drove you to embark on this path? How has your life transformed positively after initiating your strength training journey? Your narrative carries significant weight and has the potential to motivate those in your midst.

- Stay driven and establish new ambitious goals: Constantly set challenging yet attainable goals to maintain the excitement and effectiveness of your workouts. Whether it's enhancing your strength training with heavier weights, experimenting with new workout routines, or extending your exercise sessions, setting fresh objectives can rekindle your passion. Furthermore, infuse your fitness regimen with diversity and enjoyment by incorporating a range of exercises. Experiment with different fitness classes, explore varied workout equipment, or immerse yourself in outdoor pursuits such as hiking or tending to a garden.
- Overcome challenges with a positive mindset: Focus on your capabilities rather than limitations as you age. Embrace a positive mindset to tackle challenges effectively. Embrace adaptation and modification: When faced with physical constraints, know that adjustments can always be made. Additionally, collaborate with a trainer or physiotherapist to tailor exercises to your requirements. Consistency trumps perfection; hence, understand that being consistent is vital. On the other hand, it's normal to

have days off, but what matters most is getting back to your routine and staying dedicated to your objectives.

- Health and longevity: Strength training plays a major role in preventing age-related diseases and conditions. By prioritizing your fitness now, you actively lower the risk of developing diabetes, heart disease, and other chronic ailments. Moreover, regular exercise is associated with an extended lifespan. Thus, committing to your strength training regime not only increases your years on this earth but also enhances the quality of your life.

Investing in your strength training journey is a powerful commitment to self-improvement. Aging gracefully requires perseverance, dedication, and self-care. Embrace the journey, celebrate your growth, and continue pushing yourself forward. Your dedication to strength training showcases your resilience and mental fortitude. Every ounce of effort contributes to a healthier, more vibrant version of yourself. Stay resilient, stay driven, and always believe in your immense capabilities. Your future holds abundant opportunities for strength, vitality, and endless growth.

ADDITIONAL RESOURCES FOR FURTHER LEARNING AND SUPPORT

Beginning a strength training journey can ignite excitement and empowerment, particularly when equipped with the necessary resources. Discover here a selection of valuable tools to kick-start and maintain your motivation.

Books and Guides

- *Fitness After 40: How to Stay Strong at Any Age* by Vonda Wright, M.D.

It offers insights and exercises suitable for those over 40, with adaptations for different fitness levels and ages.

- *Strong Women Stay Young* by Miriam E. Nelson, Ph.D.

It focuses on the benefits of strength training for older women and provides practical routines to follow.

Online Platforms and Communities

- SilverSneakers: A popular fitness program designed for older adults, offering both in-person and online classes, including strength training, cardio, and flexibility exercises. There is a large variety of videos, for example: "Cardio exercises for heart rate recovery, 15-minute workout for arthritis, etc."

  - Website: https://www.silversneakers.com/
  - Facebook page: https://www.facebook.com/silver sneakers/
  - YouTube channel: https://www.youtube.com/@silver sneakers

- National Institute on Aging (NIA): Provides a wealth of information on physical activity and exercise for older adults, including strength training guidelines and safety tips.

  - Website: https://www.nia.nih.gov/health/exercise- physical-activity

- ElderGym: An online resource with videos, exercise routines, and tips specifically for seniors looking to improve their strength, balance, and flexibility.

- ○ Website: https://www.eldergym.com/

YouTube Channels

- HASfit: Offers a range of free workout videos, including strength training routines for seniors, with modifications for different fitness levels. They also have a playlist of videos.

  - ○ YouTube Channel: https://www.youtube.com/user/KozakSportsPerform
  - ○ Ex. YouTube Video: https://www.youtube.com/watch?v=LHx3eP93Zrg&list=PLRCgg2aTq5NUlZ6YI-lEg-T1iZgvRtYh-&index=5

- Senior Fitness with Meredith: Features a variety of exercise videos tailored for older adults, focusing on strength, balance, and flexibility.

  - ○ YouTube Channel: https://www.youtube.com/@SeniorFitnessWithMeredith

- Bob & Brad: Physical therapists who have a variety of exercise videos, as well as informative videos about your health and symptoms of health conditions to be aware of. They provide exercise videos and advice on maintaining fitness and mobility as you age, including strength training tips.

  - ○ YouTube Channel: https://www.youtube.com/user/physicaltherapyvideo

Apps and Digital Tools

- FitOn: A free app offering a variety of workout videos, including strength training sessions suitable for seniors.

  - Website: https://fitonapp.com/

- Sworkit: Provides customizable workout plans, including strength training routines, with a focus on beginner-friendly exercises.

  - Website: https://sworkit.com/

Local Resources and Support

- Community centers and gyms: Many community centers and gyms offer fitness classes specifically for seniors. They are worth visiting and it's a good idea to try out a few different places to see if they are the right fit for you.
- Personal trainers specialized in older adults: If it makes you more comfortable, think about hiring a certified personal trainer who specializes in working with older adults. They can provide you with personalized guidance, ensure that your form is correct, and help design your workout plan. It is important to look around and try a few different trainers; they must be a fit for you, and do not be afraid to say when it is not! They can provide personalized guidance and ensure you're performing exercises safely and effectively.
- Senior fitness groups: Joining local fitness groups or clubs can provide motivation, comradery, accountability, and a support net. This is, once again, where you have to try out

a variety of groups. It will not be enjoyable if you are grouped with people you do not get along with.

SUMMARY

Starting a strength training journey as a woman over 60 is a commendable step toward improving your health and well-being. Utilizing these resources can provide you with the knowledge, support, and motivation needed to create a successful and enjoyable fitness routine. Remember, it's important to consult with your health care provider before beginning any new exercise program, especially if you have any existing health conditions or concerns. With the right resources and a positive mindset, you can achieve your fitness goals and enjoy a healthier, more active lifestyle.

Glossary

Arthritis: Arthritis is when the joints get all inflamed, making them hurt and feel stiff.

Body Awareness Sense: The body telling the brain where it's at, how it's moving, and where it's going.

Bone Density: How tough and mineral-filled the bones are.

Cardiovascular Exercise: Exercises that get the heart pumping fast, like jumping jacks or running.

Chronic Illness: A long-lasting health problem that doesn't go away easily.

Electrolytes: Tiny particles in the body that carry electricity to make sure everything works right.

Estrogen: The boss lady hormone in the female body, calling the shots on periods and keeping everything in balance.

Glycogen: The snack stash your body saves for emergencies. It's quick energy waiting to be used during exercise or when you need a boost.

High-Intensity Interval Training (HIIT): Workouts that mix going all out with catching your breath. It's like sprinting hard, then walking to catch your breath before going again.

Insulin Resistance: When the body doesn't respond well to insulin, the sugar in the blood doesn't get used properly. It's like the body's cells forgetting how to open the door for sugar to come inside.

Menopause: When a woman's ovaries stop producing hormones and menstrual periods do not occur for 12 months. Menopause tends to occur around 50 years of age but differs for every individual. There are many symptoms, some more severe than others.

Multi-Frequency Segmental Devices: These cool devices shake things up by using different frequencies to analyze what your body's made of.

Muscle Mass: The amount of muscle you've got, helping you lift heavy things and stay active. The more muscle, the stronger you are!

Osteoblasts: Cells that build new bone tissue to keep the skeleton strong. These cells synthesize and secrete bone matrix and contribute in the mineralization of bone that regulates the balance of calcium and phosphate ions in creating bone.

Osteoporosis: When the bones get weak and might break easily, especially in older folks.

Progesterone: A sex hormone that is involved in pregnancy and the menstrual cycle. It helps out during pregnancy and keeps hormones balanced. It belongs to a group of steroid hormones and is created by the ovaries and the testes.

Progressive Overload: This fitness trick means gradually making workouts tougher so the muscles grow stronger.

Protein Synthesis: The body's constantly building and fixing itself with the help of proteins made through this process.

Sarcopenia: The muscle mass starts shrinking as one gets older, making it harder to move around. Sarcopenia is a musculoskeletal disease where muscle mass, strength, and performance are significantly breaking down as an individual ages—more so than normal.

Strength Training: When you lift weights or do exercises to challenge your muscles, you're doing strength training.

Testosterone: The male sex hormone that is made in the testicles. Testosterone hormone levels are important to normal male sexual development and functions. During puberty, this helps with the development of male features like body and facial hair, deeper voice, and muscle strength.

REFERENCES

Balance boards: Benefits, drawbacks, and exercises. (2021, February 24). Healthline. https://www.healthline.com/health/fitness/balance-board-exercises

Barahona-Fuentes, G., Huerta Ojeda, Á., & Chirosa-Ríos, L. (2021). Effects of training with different modes of strength intervention on psychosocial disorders in adolescents: A systematic review and meta-analysis. *International Journal of Environmental Research and Public Health, 18*(18), 9477. https://doi.org/10.3390/ijerph18189477

Berg-Hansen, P., Moen, S. T., Klyve, T. D., Gonzalez, V., Seeberg, T. M., Celius, E. G., Austeng, A., & Meyer, F. (2023). The instrumented single leg stance test detects early balance impairment in people with multiple sclerosis. *Frontiers in Neurology, 14.* https://doi.org/10.3389/fneur.2023.1227374

Benefits of branched-chain amino acid supplements for post-workout recovery. (n.d.). Camelbak. https://www.camelbak.com/blog-benefits-branched-chained-amino-acid-supplements.html

Bielecki, J. E., & Tadi, P. (2021). *Therapeutic exercise.* National Library of Medicine. https://www.ncbi.nlm.nih.gov/books/NBK555914/

Bonvissuto, D. (2018, February 26). *What medicines can cause dehydration?* WebMD. https://www.webmd.com/drug-medication/medicines-can-cause-dehydration

Castro-Sloboda, G. (n.d.). *Do ankle and wrist weights actually help your workout? Experts explain.* CNET. https://www.cnet.com/health/fitness/do-ankle-and-wrist-weights-actually-help-your-workout-experts-explain/

The contribution of drinking water to mineral nutrition in humans. (1980). In *Drinking water and health Volume 3* National Academies Press. https://www.ncbi.nlm.nih.gov/books/NBK216589/

Creatine. (2023, April 26). Cleveland Clinic. https://my.clevelandclinic.org/health/treatments/17674-creatine

Cross training. (n.d.). OrthoInfo. https://orthoinfo.aaos.org/en/staying-healthy/cross-training/

Duren, D. L., Sherwood, R. J., Czerwinski, S. A., Lee, M., Choh, A. C., Siervogel, R. M., & Chumlea, Wm. C. (2008). Body Composition Methods: Comparisons and Interpretation. *Journal of Diabetes Science and Technology, 2*(6), 1139–1146. https://doi.org/10.1177/193229680800200623

Eastman, H. (2021, July 1). *How micronutrients impact your fitness and physique.* Body

Building. https://www.bodybuilding.com/content/top-5-micronutrient-short falls.html

Elliott, B. (n.d.). *The ultimate guide to foam Rolling for recovery.* Muscle & Fitness. https://www.muscleandfitness.com/workouts/workout-tips/foam-rolling-total-body-benefits/

Fischer, K. (2022, December 22). *What is progressive overload?* WebMD. https://www.webmd.com/fitness-exercise/progressive-overload

Food as fuel before, during and after workouts. (2015, September 1). heart.org. https://www.heart.org/en/healthy-living/healthy-eating/eat-smart/nutrition-basics/food-as-fuel-before-during-and-after-workouts

Health benefits of protein powder. (2018, September 18). Medical News Today. https://www.medicalnewstoday.com/articles/323093

Healthy meal planning: Tips for older adults. (n.d.). National Institute on Aging. https://www.nia.nih.gov/health/healthy-eating-nutrition-and-diet/healthy-meal-planning-tips-older-adults

Heimlich, J. (2024, February 12). *You don't need to lift heavy weights to build bigger muscles.* GQ. https://www.gq.com/story/how-to-get-bigger-muscles

High intensity exercise vs low intensity exercise - which is best? (2021, August 16). Forth. https://www.forthwithlife.co.uk/blog/high-intensity-vs-low-intensity-exercise/

How microtears help you to build muscle mass. (n.d.). University Hospitals. https://www.uhhospitals.org/blog/articles/2018/02/microtears-and-mass

Howe, L. (2019, July 16). *A guide to assessing mobility for strength and conditioning coaches.* SimpliFaster. https://simplifaster.com/articles/mobility-assessment-guide-strength-coaches/

Improving health and preventing injury with strength training. (n.d.). Coreshorts. https://coreshorts.com/blogs/news/improving-health-and-preventing-injury-with-strength-training

LaPelusa, A., & Kaushik, R. (2022, November 14). *Physiology, proteins.* PubMed. https://www.ncbi.nlm.nih.gov/books/NBK555990/

Maximizing muscle recovery: The role of post-workout nutrition. (2023, November 27). Rupa Health. https://www.rupahealth.com/post/maximizing-muscle-recovery-the-role-of-post-workout-nutrition

Mayo Clinic Staff. (2020, October 14). *Water: How much should you drink every day?* Mayo Clinic. https://www.mayoclinic.org/healthy-lifestyle/nutrition-and-healthy-eating/in-depth/water/art-20044256

Mielgo-Ayuso, J., & Fernández-Lázaro, D. (2021). Nutrition and muscle recovery. *Nutrients, 13*(2), 294. https://doi.org/10.3390/nu13020294

Nystoriak, M. A., & Bhatnagar, A. (2018). Cardiovascular effects and benefits of exercise. *Frontiers in Cardiovascular Medicine, 5*(135). https://doi.org/10.3389/fcvm.2018.00135

Pain and injuries after exercise. (n.d.). NHS Inform. https://www.nhsinform.scot/illnesses-and-conditions/muscle-bone-and-joints/pain-and-injuries-after-exercise/

Parker, R. (2019, September 13). *How to test flexibility and balance.* Human Kinetics Blog. https://humankinetics.me/2019/09/13/how-to-test-flexibility-and-balance/

Popkin, B. M., D'Anci, K. E., & Rosenberg, I. H. (2020). Water, hydration, and health. *Nutrition Reviews, 68*(8), 439–458. PubMed Central. https://doi.org/10.1111/j.1753-4887.2010.00304.x

Resistance bands: Put some snap in your strength training. (n.d.). Cleveland Clinic. https://health.clevelandclinic.org/should-you-try-resistance-bands-for-strength-training

Robinson, K. M. (2014, July 18). *Circuit training.* WebMD. https://www.webmd.com/fitness-exercise/a-z/circuit-training

Seguin, R. A., Epping, J. N., Buchner, D. M., Bloch, R. & Nelson, M. E. (2003). *Growing stronger: Strength training for older adults.* CDC. https://www.cdc.gov/physicalactivity/downloads/growing_stronger.pdf

Senior citizen fitness test. (n.d.). Unacademy. https://unacademy.com/content/cbse-class-12/study-material/physical-education/senior-citizen-fitness-test/

7 great reasons why exercise matters. (2021, October 8). Mayo Clinic. https://www.mayoclinic.org/healthy-lifestyle/fitness/in-depth/exercise/art-20048389

Sexton, C. (n.d.). *The role of hydration in enhancing your workout performance.* One Life Fitness. https://www.onelifefitness.com/news/the-role-of-hydration-in-enhancing-your-workout-performance

Shrimanker, I., & Bhattarai, S. (2023). *Electrolytes.* StatPearls Publishing. https://www.ncbi.nlm.nih.gov/books/NBK541123/

Six minute walk test. (n.d.). Physiopedia. https://www.physio-pedia.com/Six_Minute_Walk_Test_/_6_Minute_Walk_Test

Stretching: Focus on flexibility. (2022, February 12). Mayo Clinic. https://www.mayoclinic.org/healthy-lifestyle/fitness/in-depth/stretching/art-20047931

Thompson, K. (2023, April 18). *The benefits of exercising with a stability ball.* North Central Surgical Hospital. https://northcentralsurgical.com/the-benefits-of-exercising-with-a-stability-ball/

Volpi, E., Nazemi, R., & Fujita, S. (2004). Muscle tissue changes with aging. *Current Opinion in Clinical Nutrition and Metabolic Care, 7*(4), 405–410. https://doi.org/10.1097/01.mco.0000134362.76653.b2

Walker, B. (2008, July 23). *What is interval training? | Examples of interval training.* Stretch Coach. https://stretchcoach.com/articles/interval-training/

Waldegger, S., Busch, G. L., Kaba, N. K., Zempel, G., Ling, H., Heidland, A., Häussinger, D., & Lang, F. (1997). Effect of cellular hydration on protein metabolism. *Mineral and Electrolyte Metabolism, 23*(3-6), 201–205. https://pubmed.ncbi.nlm.nih.gov/9387117/

Water and hydration: Physiological basis in adults. (n.d.). Hydration for Health. https://www.hydrationforhealth.com/en/hydration-science/hydration-lab/water-and-hydration-physiological-basis-adults/

Warm up, cool down. (2014, September 1). American Heart Association. https://www.heart.org/en/healthy-living/fitness/fitness-basics/warm-up-cool-down

What women need to know about weight training and weight gain. (n.d.). MSFIT. https://msfit.sg/blog/what-women-need-to-know-about-weight-training-and-weight-gain

Made in the USA
Middletown, DE
08 September 2024

60622601R00091